The Sweating
Sickness Epidemic

The Sweating Sickness Epidemic

Henry VIII's Great Fear

Stephen Porter

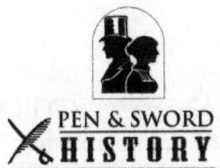

First published in Great Britain in 2023 by
Pen & Sword History
An imprint of
Pen & Sword Books Ltd
Yorkshire – Philadelphia

Copyright © Stephen Porter 2023

ISBN 978 1 39906 428 6

The right of Stephen Porter to be identified as Author of this work has been asserted by him in accordance with the Copyright, Designs and Patents Act 1988.

A CIP catalogue record for this book is
available from the British Library.

All rights reserved. No part of this book may be reproduced or transmitted in any form or by any means, electronic or mechanical including photocopying, recording or by any information storage and retrieval system, without permission from the Publisher in writing.

Typeset by Mac Style
Printed in the UK by CPI Group (UK) Ltd, Croydon, CR0 4YY.

Pen & Sword Books Limited incorporates the imprints of Atlas, Archaeology, Aviation, Discovery, Family History, Fiction, History, Maritime, Military, Military Classics, Politics, Select, Transport, True Crime, Air World, Frontline Publishing, Leo Cooper, Remember When, Seaforth Publishing, The Praetorian Press, Wharncliffe Local History, Wharncliffe Transport, Wharncliffe True Crime and White Owl.

For a complete list of Pen & Sword titles please contact

PEN & SWORD BOOKS LIMITED
47 Church Street, Barnsley, South Yorkshire, S70 2AS, England
E-mail: enquiries@pen-and-sword.co.uk
Website: www.pen-and-sword.co.uk

Or

PEN AND SWORD BOOKS
1950 Lawrence Rd, Havertown, PA 19083, USA
E-mail: Uspen-and-sword@casematepublishers.com
Website: www.penandswordbooks.com

Contents

Acknowledgements vii
Abbreviations viii

Chapter 1   The King and the Sweat   1

Chapter 2   Plague and Pestilence   11

Chapter 3   Environments   21

Chapter 4   The Sweat in Henry VII's Reign   38

Chapter 5   A Sickly Decade   52

Chapter 6   The Outbreaks of 1528 and 1529   69

Chapter 7   The Final Epidemic   86

Chapter 8   Recollections   104

Appendix 1: The Household Orders of 1539   123
Appendix 2: The Sweating Sickness in Holinshed's Chronicles   128
Notes   132
Bibliography   143
Index   149

Among the array of diseases that brought death to Tudor England, the sweating sickness stood out as truly terrifying. The speed with which it struck, its dreadful effects on its victims and the death rates that it produced, together generated a fear verging on panic when it was identified. The sweating sickness attacked the cities, towns and the countryside, not sparing the palaces. It threatened everyone, from the king in his castle to the beggars at his gates, including members of the dynasty and the political structure, the courtiers and those who ran the government, church and the law. Contemporaries could do little more than make a bolt for it, and that included the king and his closest advisors, who moved furtively in a small group from one house to another away from London.

The principal epidemics came between 1485, when it made its first appearance, and 1551, and it was confined to England and Wales, apart from one major eruption across northern Europe in 1529. Known as the English disease, this rapidly acting virus became Henry VIII's overriding fear, aggravating his well-known hypochondria and controlling his movements. Its nature, incidence and impact are examined here, in the context of Tudor England and the problems of the Henrician succession.

Acknowledgements

This book owes its existence to two Stephens: my late husband the author Stephen Porter, who wrote the text, and his friend Dr Stephen Roberts, who saw the work through to publication. As his health declined, my husband asked Dr Roberts to take on the onerous task of editing and making the manuscript fit for publication. Without a quibble, Stephen Roberts diligently set about his task and enabled this book to see the light of day. I am truly indebted to Stephen Roberts for his persistence and expertise. I am very grateful to everyone at Pen and Sword who made this book possible and for their understanding in dealing with a posthumous publication. Finally, I would like to thank the National Gallery of Art in Washington, the Wellcome Collection and the Yale Center for British Art for making so many of their images freely available.

Carolyn Porter

Abbreviations

APC	*Acts of the Privy Council*
Correspondence of Erasmus	R.A.B. Mynors, A. Dalzell and J.M. Estes, eds., *The Correspondence of Erasmus: Letters 1356 to 1534,* Toronto, University of Toronto Press, 1974 continuing
CSPD	*Calendar of State Papers, Domestic*
CSPVen	*Calendar of State Papers, Venetian*
Hall, *Chronicle*	*The Lives of the Kings. By Edward Hall* ed. C. Whibley, 2 vols. London, T.C. and E.C. Jack, 1904
L&P	*Letters and Papers, Foreign and Domestic, Henry VIII*
LMA	London Metropolitan Archives
ODNB	*Oxford Dictionary of National Biography*
TNA	The National Archives
VCH	Victoria History of the Counties of England

Chapter One

The King and the Sweat

Henry VIII's fear of the sweating sickness was so great that just the mention of it was so 'terrible and fearful to his Highness' ears that he dare in no wise approach unto the place where it is noised to have been'. That was written roughly midway through his long reign of 38 years but would have been true at any stage during his time on the throne. Of course, a monarch needed to be aware of the dangers of any disease which might bring incapacitation, even for a while, paralysing the political process, or possibly death; Henry's brother Arthur had died at the age of 15 of 'a malign vapour which proceeded from the air', which has not been identified. That may have contributed to Henry's especial fear of the sweat, which was difficult to avoid as it came on suddenly and struck down its victims quickly. Moreover, it had reputedly first arrived with his father's army in 1485 and to a remorseful person that could have been interpreted as inflicting a curse, for he had taken the throne by force from Richard III at the Battle of Bosworth. The chronicle of the Franciscan friary in London described its first onset succinctly: 'This year was a great death and hasty, called the sweating sickness'.[1]

The malady's most obvious symptom gave it that common name of 'the sweating sickness', or simply 'the sweat'. It was an affliction of early Tudor England and has vanished. Modern attempts to link it with a known disease have not been convincing and so it remains an unidentified illness, as mysterious to modern scholars as to those Tudor Englishmen, including the royal family, who could scarcely take action swiftly enough to avoid it. Suggestions made during the twentieth century were that it was an enterovirus or arbovirus, anthrax, or a hantavirus. None of these entirely fits the evidence and so the identity of this devastating disease remains unknown.[2]

According to a narrator (who has become known as the Croyland Chronicler) of Henry Tudor's brief campaign to seize the throne from Richard III, after Tudor's army had landed at Milford Haven on 7 August, the king sent to Lord Stanley, lord chamberlain of North Wales, 'requesting him without the least delay, to present himself before him at Nottingham…[but] he made an excuse that he was suffering from an attack of the sweating sickness, and could not possibly come'.[3] Stanley and his son were playing a waiting game and at that stage prevaricated, not committing themselves and their forces until the day of battle. In June that year, the York civic records mention that there was pestilence in the region, which was too early in the year for plague to have become a problem. Perhaps that was the new disease. But the simplest response was to attribute the outbreak to two of the commonest dislikes of the general population: foreigners and soldiers. Tudor's army consisted of his band of sometimes boisterous exiles, who had been based at Vannes in Brittany for over a year, professional soldiers hired in the summer of 1485 mostly from the members of the disbanded garrison of Pont L'Arche, and a force of Scottish mercenaries, perhaps 5,000 men in all. According to the chronicler Philippe de Commynes, this small army included 'three thousand of the most unruly men that could be found and enlisted in Normandy'.[4] The incubation period for the virus seems to have been around three weeks, and so if Tudor's army from Brittany had included men or camp followers who were infective, the disease would have broken out among them before the battle of Bosworth was fought on 22 August. It is inconceivable that the commanders of forces suffering from an outbreak of that kind would have offered battle, as Tudor did, and it is quite improbable that with some soldiers in the debilitated condition which it produced they would have won, against odds of three to one. Richard was killed in the battle. It therefore seems unlikely that the disease came with the mercenaries from Brittany. Its commanders had been in touch with the Stanleys after Henry had landed and the disease could have been transmitted between the two forces during that process, but even then some members of the army, which consisted of Tudor's and the Stanleys' merged forces, would have succumbed to the virus in the aftermath of the battle, as it marched from the Midlands to London with the new king.

Henry himself was in no hurry to go to London and travelled 'by easy journeys' before arriving at Shoreditch on 3 September, where he was received by the Mayor and aldermen, with trumpeters playing, and then going to St Paul's for prayers of thanksgiving and a *Te Deum*, before taking up residence at the Bishop of London's palace. He did not ride through London to the cathedral, or travel in 'any open chair or throne, but in a close chariot', which suggests a nervousness for his safety and uncertainty about Londoners' reaction to events but clearly he was not thought to be in danger from disease at that stage. The sweating sickness erupted in the City 'towards the end of September', with victims recorded around 21 September. On the 23rd the Mayor, Thomas Hill, died and his successor, Sir William Stokker, died on 28 September; four aldermen and 'many worshipful commoners' also died in the epidemic.[5] It had appeared earlier in Oxford, where an entry in the annals of Merton College stated that the disease broke out in the university 'around the end of August and the beginning of September' and that 'towards the end of September this fatal disease suddenly spread throughout the whole kingdom'.[6] The direct route from Leicestershire to the capital was along Watling Street, well to the east of Oxford, and there is no reason to think that the army deviated from the obvious course to such an extent as to have passed through the city, although a detachment may have been sent to secure it, as a strategically placed walled city.

It may be that the disease came from the Baltic or northern Germany, where the population had developed enough resistance for it not to cause high mortality, and reached England across the North Sea, making an impact during the summer. It then was transmitted by the Stanleys' forces and when it reached a virgin population in southern England it produced many deaths. Another possibility is that the disease came to England, perhaps directly to London, the country's chief trading port, from some unidentified source and as its onset roughly coincided with the arrival of armed foreigners there they were blamed and so there was no need to look further for an explanation. The accepted view was expressed by the historian John Noorthouck in 1773, that the sweating sickness 'is said to have first appeared among the troops he [Henry Tudor] brought with him from France'.[7] Shakespeare associated the disease with war, punishment and poverty. In *Measure for Measure* (1604) Mistress Overdone complains that business at her brothel is declining 'what with the war, what with the sweat, what with the gallows, and what with poverty, I am custom-shrunk'. Plague is not mentioned in that play.[8] Perhaps the sweating sickness in some form was endemic in northern France and that was the source, but the 'Picardy Sweats', which have been compared with the sweating sickness, were not identified until 1718. A direct route of infection with Tudor's army seems doubtful, if only because of the incubation period and the earlier references in the York records, although the later outbreaks could have resulted from sporadic introductions into England from France.[9]

Although it struck less frequently than did plague and carried off fewer victims, the speed of the sweat's onset and the rapidity with which its sufferers succumbed were truly frightening. Polydore Vergil, an Italian writer settled in England, described how 'A sudden deadly sweating attacked the body and at the same time head and stomach were in pain from the violence of the fever'. He wrote that this was 'a new kind of disease … a baleful affliction and one which no previous age had experienced', which produced 'a disastrous loss of life'. Thomas Forestier, a physician from Rouen in Normandy but possibly trained in Italy, who was based in London in the autumn of 1485, was so concerned about the death and distress that the new disease caused that he wrote a treatise on the subject, which he described as 'the venomous fever of pestilence' that 'vexed and troubled' not only the king and his 'great power', but also 'thy lordships and almost the middle part of thy realm'. Among the symptoms were a 'redness of the face and of all the body' produced by a skin irritation and a rash of spots, and 'a continual thirst, with a great heat and headache'. Forestier's essay was the first to deal with the subject and in it he gave space not only to the disease but also to hygiene, stressing the dangers of polluted water, foul vapours and bad air, and the benefits of clear, pure water and a good diet, while also giving some credence to astrological influences.[10] After a later outbreak, in 1551, John Caius, a physician who had trained at Padua, published a tract on the disease in which he claimed that it was an ailment 'which for the sudden sharpness and unwonted cruelness passed the pestilence'.[11]

One of the sweat's characteristics was the speed with which it killed those who were infected. Dr Caius summarised that aspect of the affliction, noting that some died 'in opening their windows, some in playing with children in their street doors; some in one hour, many in two, it destroyed; and at the longest to them that merrily dined, it gave a sorrowful supper. As it found them, so it took them; some in sleep, some in wake, some in mirth, some in care, some fasting and some full, some busy and some idle; and in one house sometime three, sometime five, sometime more, sometime all'. It was aptly named, although at first a victim, after feeling unwell, was wracked by cold shivers, with dizziness and pains in the head and neck. Only in the second phase did hot sweats and intense thirst, palpitations and delirium sweep over the sufferer, who exuded a foul-smelling perspiration, and the final stages were marked by exhaustion and an overwhelming desire to go to sleep. Giacomo Soranzo was newly arrived in England as the Venetian ambassador when the disease struck in 1551, and he described it as causing 'a most profuse sweat, which without any other indisposition seized patients by the way, and the remedies at first administered taking no effect they died in a few hours'.[12]

Not all victims displayed the symptoms in the same way, for there were 'some that sweat much, and some that sweat very little'. Either way, it was all over within a short time and the sufferers had either died or were on the road to recovery. Those who survived for 24 hours were thought to be safe. The chronicler Edward Hall wrote of those who contracted the disease that 'many died within five or six hours'. Thomas More told Erasmus, from experience in the 1517 epidemic, that 'this sweating sickness is fatal only on the first day'.[13] According to Elizabeth, Duchess of Norfolk, in 1528, 'about 12 or 16 hours is the greatest danger', while Caius thought that the crucial period was the first 12 to 14 hours. Edward VI's opinion as to timing, from the victims of the 1551 epidemic, was that 'if one took cold, he died within three hours, and if he escaped, it held him but nine hours, or ten at the most'.[14] The death rate was very high and only a fortunate few survived, for 'all alike died, either as soon as the fever began or not long after, so that of all the persons infected scarcely one in a hundred escaped death'.[15]

After the initial epidemic in 1485, outbreaks occurred in England in 1506, 1508, 1511, 1517, 1518, 1528, 1529, 1533 and, after a long interval, in 1551, which was the last widespread appearance of the disease. There may have been more outbreaks. When Erasmus wrote to Cardinal Wolsey's physician in 1515 he mentioned that 'I am frequently astonished and grieved to think how it is that England has been now for so many years troubled by a continual pestilence, especially by a deadly sweat, which appears in a great measure to be peculiar to your country'.[16] Caius pointed out that when Englishmen fled abroad to avoid the sweat, to Calais, Antwerp and other places in Brabant, 'only our countrymen were sick, and none others, except one or two'. He noted that 'this disease is almost peculiar unto us English men, and not common to all men' and that 'because it first began in England, it was named in other countries, the English sweat'; this he attributed to 'the English diet'.[17] Indeed, the disease had already come to be known as the English Sweat, *Sudor Anglicus*; Thomas Hubertus contracted the disease, which he described as 'the evil illness which men call the English sweat, since it came from England'. No convincing evidence has been found that the disease spread to Scotland, Wales or Ireland, although an outbreak in Ireland in 1492 has been postulated. Brian Tuke commented that in France and Flanders it was called the king of England's sickness, 'and is not thought much of there'. He believed that although people travelled between Calais, then an English town, and nearby Gravelines, the disease was not transmitted between the two places.[18] The only major epidemic of the disease on the continent came in 1529, when it struck much of northern Europe and Germany, penetrating as far south as Austria and Switzerland.

Remedies were suggested and applied. The Duchess of Norfolk believed that those who died did so because of lack of proper nursing, which should be carried out 'as well as is possible after the temperate fashion'. She also recommended that the victims should be kept in bed for 24 hours and 'take little or no sustenance or drink until 16 hours be past'. To those who showed a swollen stomach she gave 'setwell [valerian] to eat, the which drives it away from the stomach'. She also dosed the sufferers with 'Vinegar, wormwood, rosewater, and crumbs of brown bread [which] is very good and comfortable to put in a linen cloth to smell unto your nose, so that it touch not your visage [face]'.[19] Fasting was recommended by some writers; one wrote that the victims should 'neither to drink nor eat to noon'. In Vergil's opinion, patients should go to bed, fully dressed, and remain there for 24 hours, not allowed food but permitted 'enough of his usual drink warmed to quench his thirst'. If the patient could not sweat, despite the amount of covering, 'then heat two or three bricks or tiles in the fire and warm them in a moist linen cloth, and lay them by his sides in the bed, and that shall cause him to sweat'. A most important aspect of the nursing was to ensure that the patient should remain fully covered, with not even a limb exposed outside the bedclothes for coolness 'for this is fatal'. Jean du Bellay, the French ambassador in England, believed that 'if a man only put his hand out of bed during twenty-four hours, it becomes as stiff as a pane of glass'. He wrote that the disease 'is the easiest in the world to die of'. Of course, it was a simple thing for those who were well to make suggestions that were to be applied, by fearless apothecaries and nurses, to those who were sick. As Erasmus recognised in his *Adages* of the early sixteenth century, 'when we are well we find it easy to give good advice to the sick', which was probably the dramatist John Lyly's source for his observation in *Galatea*, performed in 1580, that 'in health it is easy to counsel the sick, but it's hard for the sick to follow wholesome counsel'.[20]

Not surprisingly, some of those who were at the sweating stage tried to push away the bedclothes to get relief from the overwhelming heat, but that was thought to be dangerous and extra bedding should be added to maintain the high temperature, until the patient had sweated out the disease. The aim was that the patient would 'perspire gently and naturally'. The chances of recovery could be good 'if the patient were kept in an equal temper, both for clothes, fire, and drink moderately warm, with temperate cordials, whereby nature's work were neither irritated by heat nor turned back by cold'. Slightly different advice was given in 1528 for Lord Darcy's household, where 30 people were 'all in peril'. A drink was to be prepared and heated 'and so let the patient drink it, and keep him well, neither over hot nor over cold, but whole in his arms and feet, and let him keep him by taking clothes off him by little and little, till he be dried up, and let him use wholesome meats, and by the grace of God he shall not perish'. Whatever nursing was applied, 'the greatest surety is in any wise to keep your bed 24 hours'. But a sluggish response or failure to recognise the nature of the sickness in time could thwart the best nursing care and 'infinite persons died suddenly of it, before the manner of the cure and attendance was known'.[21] Patients who were being nursed and had passed the worst were not out of danger; their nurses needed to be vigilant and stay with the patient throughout the 24 hours. According to Caius, they should 'endeavour themselves to be handsome and diligent about us, to serve us readily at all turns, and never to leave us during four and twenty hours, but to look well unto us, that neither we cast off our clothes, nor thrust out hand or foot, during the space of the said four and twenty hours'. He believed that some died after the crisis seemed to have passed, through over-confidence that they were on the way to recovery, or because of 'negligence in attendance, when they think no necessity. Whereby it is proved that without doubt, the handsome diligence, or careless negligence, is the saving, or casting away of many'.[22] One of the nurses' duties was to keep the patient awake during the early stages, overcoming a craving to sleep. Nursing care was so expensive, and the nurses took such risks, that when an epidemic struck and many victims required care at the same time, then only the patients from wealthy families could obtain the nursing that they required. The Duchess of Norfolk offered Wolsey the services of two nurses if he should catch the sweat, and they would keep him 'as well as is possible after the temperate fashion'.[23] The various medicines, too, would be dear, because they used expensive ingredients, as well as some fanciful ones, such as 'half a nutshell full of unicorn's horn scraped small' and 'powder of unicorn's horns'. Some were designated with names which were designed to give their users confidence in their efficacy, such as 'The king's medicine for the pestilence' and a 'proved medicine against the pestilence, called the philosopher's egg'.[24]

Care was still required when the sweating was over. One recommendation went into detail about this: 'as the patient sweats, to wipe away the sweat from his body downward with hot dry cloths, and his sweating being ended you must shift his shirt and all the bedding with fresh warm clothes, using him very warm from any cold taking in the meantime, and let him sit well wrapped by a warm fire while his bed is preparing to be made'. While the patient was recuperating 'he shall eat no flesh nor drink wine for the space of one week', and another concoction was to be given to him. Getting hot again was to be avoided and so the recovering patient should not take baths for they 'open the pores of the body, and make the venomous airs to enter, and destroy the lively spirits in man, and enfeeble the body'. Food that was inclined to create body heat, such as garlic, onions and leeks, was to be avoided, and the patient should eat little meat except 'chickens sodden with water, or fresh fish roasted to eat with vinegar. Pottage of almonds is good, and for drink tisane [barley water], or in the heat small ale. If he wishes wine, give him vinegar and water; white wine is better than red'. Whether anyone was able to follow the recommendations in the short time available, or be so well prepared as to have the ingredients to hand, may be doubted, but the disease was widespread and alarming enough for detailed remedies to be devised. To nurse a victim by provoking a sweat had to overcome the current practice for treatment of the sick for other diseases, for current medical opinion opposed the opening of the pores in the skin, which 'makes the venomous airs to enter, and destroys the lively spirits in man, and enfeebles the body'.[25] That same logic was applied to the orientation of buildings and their windows, with the preference that they should face the cool north, not the warm air from the south.

Treatment of the victims did not lessen the incidence of the disease. Caius was prepared to attribute people's vulnerability to their lifestyle: 'they which had this sweat sore with peril or death, were either men of wealth, ease, and welfare, or of the poorer sort such as were idle persons, good ale drinkers, and Tavern haunters'. His reasoning was that excessive eating and drinking without physical labour to absorb the intake caused unhealthy matter to accumulate, which the disease seized on. In his own words, 'great welfare of the one sort, and large drinking of the other, heaped up in their bodies much evil matter: by their ease and idleness, could not waste and consume it'.[26] Not all of those who sweated were infected, according to Brian Tuke, and he suggested 'that the moisture of years past hath so altered the nature both of our meats and bodies to moist humours, as disposes us to sweat'.[27] Those who were moderate in their eating and drinking were less likely to contract the disease, so that someone who wished to be 'free from sweat, must keep a pure and clean diet, and then he shall be sure'. Imperfections of the air were also partly responsible for the onset of the disease, for some reason 'all the evil air [is] apt to this disease'. Francis Bacon wrote that the sweat was due to 'a malignity in the constitution of the air, gathered by the predisposition of the seasons', which he thought explained the disease's sudden appearance and equally abrupt vanishing, which were so distinct that contemporaries were able to date them to within a day or two.[28]

Chapter Two

Plague and Pestilence

The sweat was not the sole medical source of Henry VIII's anxiety, or that of his subjects. There were many diseases for the king and his court to be apprehensive of, indeed a veritable cocktail of ailments, some fatal, some debilitating, which could lay the king low and paralyse the workings of the political system. They included unspecified fevers and agues, and contemporaries were often rather loose with their descriptions and identifications of the maladies around them.

A new disease of a venereal nature appeared in southern Europe in the last decade of the fifteenth century and became known as the 'Neapolitan sickness' or the French Pox, *Mal Francese*. It erupted in Italy in 1496 and, in a typical case of holding soldiers responsible for the appearance of a disease, was blamed by the Italians on the French armies which had invaded two years earlier, while the French attributed the outbreak to voyagers returning to Naples after the discovery of the Americas. It did not go away after its initial identification and its transmission, as with other maladies, was thought to be assisted by the movement of armies during the campaigns of the French army in Italy. The French king, Charles VIII, who commanded the army, was said to have been a victim, for he had 'a violent, hideous and abominable sickness by which he was harrowed, and several of his number, who returned to France, were most painfully afflicted by it'.[1]

England was free from military activity in the early sixteenth century, but mercenary soldiers travelled to and from the continental armies and London was a recruiting ground for professional soldiers. The city did not escape newly arrived infectious diseases, as well as those which were endemic. In 1540 surgeons in London were reproved for treating in their houses 'diseased persons as be infected with the pestilence, great pocks, and such other contagious infirmities', because they also cut hair, washed and shaved their customers on the premises, 'which is very perilous for infecting the Kings people resorting to their shoppes and houses'. By contrast, leprosy had afflicted European populations throughout the medieval period with a foul skin disorder; it is identifiable in accounts from the third century BC and the pandemic which followed probably peaked in Europe in the thirteenth and fourteenth centuries. It became less common after the Black Death, although contemporaries remained wary of it and continued to make provision for lepers outside cities and towns, to keep its victims, who were social outcasts, as far away as possible from the rest of the population, while within reach of charity. London's attitude to the disease and its victims seems to have been ambivalent. Its leper houses were around the City but outside it, for safety, and the official rule, expressed in 1472, was that the gatekeepers 'should be sworn to prevent lepers entering the City' and that annually a proclamation should be issued that 'no leper nor any person infected with the same sickness of leper enter or come within the liberty of this City of London upon pain of losing of his horse if he come riding on horseback and of his gown or upper garment of his body'. On the other hand, four years later Dame Alice Wych, widow of Sir Hugh Wych, alderman and former mayor, in her will bequeathed £1 each to three of the houses.[2]

Other ailments afflicted the population of Europe intermittently, without leaving much of a trace in the records. When he was in Basel in May 1518, Erasmus reported that 'a new kind of plague is spreading throughout Germany, which attacks a great many people'. Although that was a year when the sweating sickness struck in England, there was no suggestion that it was in any way a related disease. The symptoms were not at all similar, being 'coughs, headache, and internal pains', in some cases accompanied by delirium. Erasmus believed that 'it has killed many people but generally let the majority go free'.[3]

Of the many sicknesses of the period, plague was the most devastating and was the most virulent and harmful epidemic disease, from the Black Death in the late 1340s until the Great Plague in the mid-1660s, and the most destructive of life. It struck frequently in the fifteenth century and outbreaks continued through the sixteenth and culminated in four major epidemics in the seventeenth century. It could not be confused with the sweating sickness, which displayed quite different symptoms in the victims, and contemporaries were sure from the outset that the new disease was not the plague, or a variation of it. Plague was distinguishable from fevers and when 'the tokens, tumours, or carbuncle do appear, there is no cause of suspicion or doubt of the disease', while sweating sickness was described as a fever which produced 'an extreme sweat' and left 'no carbuncle, no purple or livid spots'.[4] The seasonality of deaths also helped to identify plague, for it was a disease of the summer and early autumn, with July, August and September the peak months for mortality from the disease, while the winter months were almost plague free.

For all its destructiveness, killing roughly three-quarters of those infected, plague was survivable by those who were able to move away. They included members of the nobility, gentry, senior churchmen, prosperous merchants and others who were well enough off to have an alternative place to go to when epidemic disease struck, but the vast majority could not afford to move away, or had no place where they would be welcome. Indeed, the disease came to be thought of as one which afflicted the poor, who had no means of taking evasive action. Henry's courtiers would have been acutely aware of its progress during a year when it was claiming victims, but it could be avoided because its patterns, seasonality and characteristics were known, and they were aware when it spread to nearby regions, so that they could put measures in place or simply move away in time. Those procedures could be cruel indeed. On at least two occasions, at Calais in 1532 and at Windsor Castle in 1540, the king ordered that those displaying plague symptoms should be taken from their beds, placed outside and left there, presumably based on the logic that the foul vapours supposedly emanating from the victims would not enter the buildings, which would safeguard their households.

In contrast to the sweating sickness, the plague bacillus is available to scientists and its characteristics have been analysed and its history traced. There have been three pandemics. The first began in the mid-sixth century in Ethiopia, reached Egypt in 540 and Constantinople in 541. Justinian I became emperor of the eastern Roman empire in 527 and during his reign the plague struck, not just the empire but most of the continent. It recurred intermittently thereafter for more than 200 years and has been known as the Plague of Justinian, reaching Scandinavia in the north and as far west as Ireland. The chronicler Procopius reported the major events of the reign from the perspective of Constantinople and described the nature of the disease, the sufferings of the victims, and the breakdown of normal social and administrative patterns, including the burial of the dead. He was so horrified by what he saw and heard that he feared that it was an illness 'by which the whole human race came near to be annihilated'.

From the mid-eighth century, Europe did not suffer from further eruptions of plague for 600 years; its absence meant that the population had no resistance to the bacterium, nor any knowledge of the form and pattern of the disease. The second pandemic began in central Asia, probably in the 1320s, and by the spring of 1346, it had reached the region between the Caspian Sea and southern Russia. From there it spread across the Black Sea to Constantinople and then on into the Mediterranean. From the autumn of 1347 North Africa and the Middle East were infected and over the next six years plague engulfed almost all of Europe, killing perhaps 50 to 60 per cent of its population, according to modern assessments. Plague outbreaks recurred frequently but irregularly over the following centuries, moving along the trade routes, both by sea and overland. Between 1536 and 1670 a plague epidemic struck western Europe on average every 15 years. It continued in the Mediterranean basin until the 1830s, although never again was it to afflict the whole continent in one devastating outbreak, as it had done in the mid-fourteenth century. But the virulence of the disease was not diminished and in some outbreaks, the proportion of the population that died was as great as during that initial outbreak.

The third pandemic began in Yunnan province in south-west China around 1860 and in 1894 there was a plague epidemic in Canton which was so devastating that the local administration was unable to record the number of victims. It then dispersed through south Asia and to Africa and both North and South America: after reaching San Francisco in 1900 it has since extended across roughly one-third of the North American continent, observed and treated, but still spreading inexorably eastwards. Australia was infected at much the same time and outbreaks there occurred between 1900 and 1925. Plague epidemics continued across much of the world through the twentieth century, with increased incidence where civil government was fractured, such as during the wars in Indo-China, and it is still present in every continent except Europe and Antarctica, its name a byword for uncontrolled disease, provoking fear and loathing.

The plague bacillus, *Yersinia pestis*, was isolated in the 1890s and the means of transmission was discovered in the following decade. Research during the terrible outbreak in India showed that it was transmitted by rats' fleas, which are parasites of the black rat. As a flea sucks blood it squirts saliva containing an anti-coagulant into the bite; the ingested blood from the host rat does not pass directly into the flea's stomach but is held initially in the proventriculus, the organ at the entrance to the stomach. If it is feeding from an infected rat, the bacilli pass with the blood and if the flea becomes infective the bacilli multiply to such an extent that they block the proventriculus. When the rat dies the flea requires another host, usually another rat or, as the rat population is killed off by the disease, it transfers to a human. When the flea again attempts to feed, the passage of blood into its stomach is obstructed by the blocked proventriculus. Unable to ingest the blood, the 'blocked' flea becomes ravenous and persists with its efforts to eat, to the point where the blood is regurgitated with the saliva, thereby carrying the plague bacilli into the bite in the skin of its human host. That process transfers the disease from rat to man, but in doing so ends the process, for the flea starves to death.

Even where the bacillus is present, the host populations of rats and their fleas need to be large enough for an epidemic to develop. In the microclimates provided by a rat's nest, stocks of grain, or textiles, which hold residual heat beyond the peak temperatures of the summer months, fleas can live for up to a year and survive cold weather, especially in nests within human dwellings or outhouses. The human flea, *Pulex irritans*, probably was also a carrier once an epidemic was under way. It is capable of being infected with *Yersinia pestis* and among its wide range of hosts are domesticated animals, including dogs, cats and pigs, so that plague spread quickly and social and economic contacts aided the diffusion of the disease.

Within the twenty-first century, ancient DNA (aDNA) analysis of dental pulp removed from skeletons in former plague burial sites in south-west France, north Italy, the Netherlands, central Germany and, in England, Hereford, Lincolnshire and London has confirmed that *Yersinia pestis* was the cause of the three pandemics. All tested positive for *Yersinia pestis*, including the skeletons from the Black Death burial grounds at Charterhouse Square and East Smithfield, and from the Great Plague of 1665 in the cemetery of Bethlehem Hospital, off Bishopsgate. *Yersinia pestis* has three subtypes: the Plague of Justinian was caused by the subtype *Antiqua*, the second pandemic by *Mediaevalis* and the third by *Orientalis*.

Without such science, explanations had to be offered by society's leaders, to divert any potential reactions against them by the populace for failing to recognise or confront the causes of an epidemic. The church's response to the catastrophic onset of the Black Death was to assert that the scourge was divine punishment for sin. It manifested God's wrath with a sinful mankind and could only be halted with the identification and then eradication of the behaviour which had prompted such an awful punishment. Expiatory services and penitential processions, organised and led by the clergy, were held and church attendance was urged so that the worshippers could take the sacraments; people were also encouraged to go on pilgrimages to holy places, as well as to examine their own lives and reform them in line with the church's teaching. Heresies were to be identified and rooted out, which led to the persecution of minorities such as the Jews. New diseases were swiftly associated with particular sins; in 1496 the Diet of Worms pronounced that the French pox was the result of excessive blasphemy.[5] In the event of an epidemic the saints were implored to intercede so that the disease would be halted by divine sanction and the survivors spared from further punishment. Some saints were particularly revered for their influence in plague times, especially Saint Sebastian and, from the mid-fifteenth century, Saint Roch. Although prayers, intercessions and penitential processions failed to halt the spread of epidemics or the return of deadly diseases, the clergy's codes of conduct for such tragic times were continued and apparently not rejected by the populace as useless.

Nor were the explanations of astrologers rejected. Their contribution to the explanation for plague was put forward during the Black Death when, in 1348, members of the University of Paris's prestigious medical faculty pointed out that at one o'clock in the afternoon on 20 March 1345 there had been a conjunction of Saturn, Jupiter and Mars. A conjunction of Saturn and Jupiter was held to bring death and depopulation, while Jupiter, as a warm and humid planet, drew up foul vapours from earth and water, and Mars was a very hot and dry planet and so set fire to the vapours. The great heat and dampness favoured pestilential vapours, which were a likely cause of the plague. Their report became widely accepted, not least because the faculty was the most distinguished of the six principal medical faculties in Europe. Yet it could be argued that no planetary conjunction lasted more than two years and, as the epidemic had continued beyond that, perhaps it was not the true cause.

Another long-standing belief, also going back to the Black Death, was that the appearance of plague was directly connected with society's excesses. Moralists had linked its reprehensible behaviour with over-indulgent dining, with rich fare consumed in quantities that verged on gluttony, and showy finery in houses and, more especially, clothing. Surely this was the sin of pride and reflected social climbing, with groups and individuals acting above their station by indulging in conspicuous consumption, rather than living an 'upright life'. The economic impact of the loss of population in the Black Death and the inflow to England from France of fine goods and wealth, from ransoms and plunder, during the first phase of the Hundred Years War, which saw almost unbroken English military successes, benefited some who had not enjoyed wealth before and who now wished to establish their newfound social status in their fashions, diets, houses and households. Rapid social mobility was not a characteristic of medieval England and when it became apparent it was deplored. For a description of Britain, published in 1480, William Caxton took as his source a fourteenth-century account. Summarising the characteristics of the English, he wrote that 'they despise what is theirs and praise what belongs to others, and are scarcely ever pleased or content with their own condition. Whatever rightly befits and appertains to others they will gladly appropriate to themselves. This is why a yeoman dresses like a squire, a squire like a knight, a knight like a duke and a duke like a king'. Then there were those 'belonging to no rank themselves' who wished to 'emulate all walks of life … willing to take on any rank' and giving themselves the appearance of 'minstrels and heralds; great orators in speech; gluttons in eating and drinking; hucksters and tavern-keepers in amassing wealth; distinguished men in dress … and owning to being churchmen only when it comes to clerical privileges and income'.[6] Abstinence and self-denial were recommended.

Thomas More's *Utopia* of 1516 describes an ideal and well-regulated commonwealth, in a literary device adopted in order to criticise aspects of English society. One of his characters makes a connection between poverty and expensive tastes: 'Servants, tradesmen, even farm-labourers, in fact all classes of society are recklessly extravagant about clothes and food. Then think how many brothels there are, including those that go under the names of wine-taverns or alehouses. Think of the demoralizing games people play – dice, cards, backgammon, tennis, bowls, quoits – what are they but quick methods of wasting a man's money, and sending him straight off to become a thief?' In his view, expensive tastes led to crime rather than divine punishment through diseases. But that reflected the thinking of the humanist circle to which More belonged rather than the ideas of the general population.[7]

To check such misplaced ambitions successive governments issued orders to regulate consumption, even to the point of specifying how many dishes of meat and fish could be served daily and fixing the maximum that could be spent on specified items by stipulated groups. The first such so-called sumptuary legislation was passed in Edward III's reign and, although those laws surely were unenforceable, they were repeated and renewed thereafter, through the fifteenth and sixteenth centuries. They were not tied specifically to outbreaks of epidemic diseases but reflected the fears of those who deplored excess and were afraid that it would provoke divine punishment. Somewhat ironically, the Black Death and the easy-going and lively atmosphere at Edward III's court had seen the introduction of fresh and, as some said, daring fashions; closely-cut gowns for women and tight hose for men which left little to the imagination and disgusted those who decried society's overindulgences. The sumptuary legislation attempted to deal with those evils, but other rules were required to achieve the cleanliness and orderliness that were also needed to appease the divine wrath.

Whatever steps were taken, they were not enough to assuage Henry VIII's concerns. Moving away when the sweat suddenly threatened was not so easy as it was when a plague epidemic developed, hence the king's great fear. But his anxious reaction to disease belied his character as a brave man skilled in the military arts, inordinately fond of hunting and, in the first half of his reign, a participant in the dangerous rough and tumble of jousts and tournaments. Henry presented himself as a chivalric king, reviving the cult of courtliness that had been promoted by Edward IV, although his father had been less attracted by it. In truth, the age of chivalry had passed and combats between knights as training for actual warfare were long out-of-date in the age of gunpowder projectiles. But jousts and tournaments kept the image alive and under Henry's patronage, 24 tournaments were held in the 1510s, before the number declined, as the king grew older, to just four in the 1540s. Henry was over six feet tall and well-built, was athletic and active and certainly did not lack courage. Nor was he deterred by accidents which could have caused him injury or even led to his death. During a tilt in 1524, the Duke of Suffolk charged the king while his visor was up 'so that his face was clean naked'; his lance 'struck the king on the brow right under the defence of the headpiece', just inches from his eye. The king accepted the blame for what had been no less than a brush with death; had a splinter hit him in the eye it surely would have proved fatal. In the following year he muffed an attempt at crossing a ditch with a pole while out on a hawking expedition: 'the pole broke, so that if one Edmond Mody, a footman, had not leapt into the water, and lift up his head, which was fast in the clay, he had been drowned'.[8] In undertaking such exploits he was taking chances with the Tudor dynasty's future as well as his own life, for he had no male heir. The only son that he and Queen Katherine produced had died in infancy and their daughter Mary was therefore heir to the throne, but a queen regnant was not a prospect which appealed to the nobility, nor could they imagine the possibility, for during the long years of the Plantagenet dynasty England had been ruled only by kings. It was therefore in the interests of the senior nobility that the king should be kept safe during epidemics and perhaps that measures should be put in place to protect both him and them.

Henry could not have avoided an awareness of plague in the family. His paternal grandmother, Margaret Beaufort, had lost her husband, Edmund Tudor, to the disease when she was pregnant with the future Henry VII. In a message to Erasmus, Henry wrote that 'it is right for mortals to submit to whatever pleases Heaven'.[9] That expression of conventional piety verged on resignation, if not fatalism, that would produce acceptance of divine chastisement rather than regulation, which could be interpreted as an attempt to thwart the divine will.

Chapter Three

Environments

Cities and towns were not chosen as places of refuge from disease when an epidemic struck: country houses and mansions offered greater safety. Access to them could be controlled and they could be built or modified in accordance with current thinking on air flow and temperatures. Conditions around the court were not encouraging for those who thought that putrefying matter and corrupt air, caused by stagnant water in pools, lakes or wells, or by decaying material in dark and dank places, provided the conditions for diseases. Filthiness and pestilential air had to be avoided through cleanliness, in public places such as the streets, squares and markets, in houses, inns and alehouses, and wherever there was standing water. In Thomas More's ideal *Utopia* there were 'special places outside the town where all blood and dirt are first washed off in running water' and it was forbidden 'to bring anything dirty or unhygienic inside the town, for fear of polluting the atmosphere and so causing disease'.[1]

Medical practice was based on the theories of Galen, and scarcely deviated from his principles. He was a court physician in second-century Rome, who believed that disease resulted from an imbalance of the four humours in the body: blood, phlegm, choler and melancholy. The imbalance was caused by the corruption of the air from 'a putrid exhalation' produced by rotting matter and, during the summer months, emissions from stagnant water, such as that in marshes and ponds, which were the result of a particular conjunction of the planets. The practical steps applied to reduce the incidence of plague and other diseases therefore corresponded to, and probably derived from, Galenic theory. Galen also pronounced that an individual's health was affected by the planets and signs of the zodiac, with each planet influencing a part of the body, and their arrangement therefore determined a person's well-being. A doctor needed to know his patient's exact time and place of birth before proceeding to diagnosis and treatment.

According to the Galenic, and therefore English, view, damp rural air was as insalubrious as were urban conditions. In England, the Fens, Somerset Levels and such marshy regions as south Essex, along the Thames estuary, had such environments but micro-climates elsewhere could also pose a danger, which John Caius summarised as being in 'close, and unstirred air, and therefore putrified or corrupt'.[2] Human exhalations were also thought to be a threat, especially where people gathered in a crowd. Gentlemen and ladies who could afford the spices and aromatic herbs required carried pomanders full of such ingredients, which they held to their faces to ward off the evil smells and dangerous exhalations. Cardinal Thomas Wolsey, the king's chief minister, was in the habit of carrying 'a very fair orange', from which the inside had been taken out and replaced by 'the part of a sponge, wherein was vinegar and other confections against the pestilent airs. This he most commonly smelt unto, when passing among the press or else when he was pestered with many visitors'.[3]

Erasmus was always alert to unhealthy environments and the risk of maladies, and he was uneasy with the English climate, objecting indignantly in 1515 that 'The common people laugh at you if you complain of a cloudy or foggy day'. He wrote that 'if ever I entered a room which had not been occupied for some months, I was sure to take a fever'. He complained that in England 'The floors are in general laid with white clay, and are covered with rushes, occasionally removed, but so imperfectly that the bottom layer is left undisturbed, sometimes for twenty years, harbouring expectorations, vomitings, the leakage of dogs and men, ale-droppings, scraps of fish, and other abominations not fit to be mentioned. Whenever the weather changes, a vapour is exhaled, which I consider very detrimental to health … I am confident the island would be much more salubrious if the use of rushes were abandoned.'

Erasmus wanted officers appointed for public places 'to see the streets cleaned from mud and urine, and the suburbs kept in better order'.[4]

Andreas Franciscius, an Italian visitor to England in 1497, also commented on the state of the streets, which were 'so badly paved' that with all the water, from carriers' carts and the rain, 'of which there is a great deal in this island', there was formed 'a vast amount of evil-smelling mud ... which does not disappear quickly but lasts a long time, in fact nearly the whole year round'. The citizens 'in order to remove this mud and filth from their boots, are accustomed to spread fresh rushes on the floors of all houses, on which they clean the soles of their shoes when they come in'. He commented that the practice was done not only by Londoners 'but also by the rest of the island's inhabitants, who, it seems, suffer from similar trouble by mud'. In discussing the sweating sickness in 1485, Thomas Forestier complained that the Londoners' habits of throwing carrion into the streets, leaving their privies dirty, and using tainted water were a source of disease. He blamed great moistness in the air and 'stinking vapours', dead animals and 'stinking waters' as causes of putrefaction which corrupted the air 'and so our bodies are infected'.[5]

In fact, the streets in London were not only paved but they and private premises were kept under surveillance for what may be termed anti-social conditions. In 1523 several defective pavements were reported, as well as premises which could cause a fire risk. Lack of ventilation was noticed: 'Three Nunnys Alley lacks a draught'; there was a 'noisome and dangerous draught in Thomas Howell's house'; in Thrum's Alley were 'draughts noisome and dangerous, as a child was lately drowned there'; tenements belonging to the Tilers' Company hall were reported to be 'very noisome for lack of draughts'; and in the aptly named Scolding Alley was 'a noisome goose house'. Use of the word 'noisome' expressed smelliness but also stagnant air, and in the context 'drowned' may have meant suffocated. Those detailed defects were noticed and reported despite the concentration of buildings in the centre of the city. Local administration was carried out by the overlapping jurisdictions of ward, parish, precinct and livery company, all of which gave attention to environmental conditions. There were 111 parishes in the City and 242 precincts, and so administration was carried out in small units, with a high proportion of householders serving as one of the local officials at some stage.

Erasmus subscribed to the opinion that windows and doors should face north and be open to the air. That was all very well for country houses and those standing on open ground, but of course, could not be achieved in an urban environment. A fresher aspect was required because: 'Englishmen's chambers are built in such a way as to admit of no ventilation. Then a great part of the walls of the house is occupied with glass casements, which admit light, but exclude the air, and yet they let in the draught through holes and corners, which is often pestilential and stagnates there'. He would have preferred it if the rooms 'were built in such a way as to be exposed to the sky on two or three sides, and all the windows so built as to be opened or closed at once; and so completely closed as not to admit the foul air through chinks; for as it is beneficial to health to admit the air, so is it equally beneficial at times to exclude it'.[6] Thomas More also favoured the 'sweet fresh air' of the countryside, contrasting it with the oppressively closed surroundings in the city. He complained that 'even houses block out from us I know not how large a measure of the light, and do not permit us to see the heavens. And the round horizon does not limit the air but the lofty roofs'.[7]

As the ex-Carthusian monk Andrew Boorde travelled in Europe he noted details of the language, culture, diet, clothing and weather of the regions through which he passed, while maintaining his interest in plague. Boorde was prepared to be flexible, but was held in by Galenic tradition and, for all his experience and observations, his was the conventional view that diseases were spread in corrupt air: 'There is nothing, except poison, that doth putrify or doth corrupt the blood of men, as doth a corrupt and contagious air'. The precautions taken were to close both the doors and windows of houses which were infected and the occupants were not to be allowed out to visit anyone, or even to go to church or to market, in case they should infect those who were 'clean without infection'. He included the stern warning that 'A man cannot be too aware, nor can keep himself too well from this sickness, for it is so vehement and so parlous, that the sickness is taken with the savour of a man's clothes the which hath visited the infectious house, for the infection will lie and hang long in clothes'. Those who remained in an infected community should daily burn in their houses juniper, rosemary, rushes, bay leaves or marjoram, frankincense or bengauyn (an aromatic resin-like substance), preferably in the morning and evening, and to ensure that the air circulated within doors a fire should be kept burning in their chambers 'of clear burning wood or charcoal without smoke'. His further advice was to 'beware of taking any cold, use temperate meats and drink, and beware of wine, beer and cider', and he warned: 'use no gross meats, but those the which be light of digestion'. Erasmus had also recommended 'more moderation in diet, and especially in the use of salt meats'. Erasmus had pondered on a possible connection between salt fish, if kept too long, and outbreaks of the sweating sickness.[8]

Many travellers across northern Europe were destined for London. London's economy attracted merchants and traders from overseas. In 1497 Franciscus wrote that 'Merchants not only from Venice but also Florence and Lucca, and many from Genoa and Pisa, from Spain, Germany, the Rhine valley and other countries meet here to handle business with the utmost keenness, having come from different parts of the world'.[9] The city had recovered from the economic malaise of the middle of the century and by the 1480s was leaving its rivals far behind, despite a high mortality rate, which was common in late medieval cities. The turnover of population there made it vulnerable to new illnesses. Diseases travelled with people, along the trade routes and regular connections between places, for commerce, pilgrimage and for those who were migrating, internally or to another country. Those migrating to a new place were generally young people and as they travelled, as well as on their arrival, they were exposed to a veritable cocktail of diseases from which they had little or no resistance. In fifteenth-century England those who sought to improve their lot through work or the patronage of senior figures were attracted primarily to London, as the largest and by far the wealthiest city, the seat of government and the court, the focus of the professions, industry and trade, both domestic and overseas; it was a bustling, growing city attracting those who were industrious, clever and ambitious. Migrants also arrived from northern Europe, especially the Low Countries, who were generally described as 'Flemish', and France, and merchants were drawn there to trade in English goods, especially its fine wool. English pilgrims most commonly visited Compostela, in north-west Spain, Rome and, much further afield, Jerusalem.

Those who landed at Dover or Sandwich made their way to Canterbury before setting off for London. Along the way from the city, they would have mingled with the pilgrims who had been to Thomas à Becket's shrine at Canterbury, one of the two most visited shrines in the country, the other being at Walsingham in Norfolk. Along the way they would have formed into groups, for company and for safety against robbers, arriving at hostelries together and crowding them; English inns were no less airless than their continental counterparts. Other shrines drew pilgrims in relatively large numbers. Another group which was on the move consisted of the students at Oxford and Cambridge, the only two universities. They were not large groups, compared with the numbers after the late sixteenth-century expansion, but they were drawn from across the country and travelled to and from their university seasonally. Those who studied at Cambridge ran the distinct risk of contracting the 'Cambridge Sweat', which seemed to strike almost annually. Certainly, the city's cold and damp climate was not conducive to good health and between 1510 and 1550 an epidemic struck the city on average every three years. Oxford, too, suffered from a reputation as being unhealthy and in the late fifteenth and early sixteenth centuries recorded twice as many deaths as births, with relatively high numbers of burials in the late summer months, when epidemics were most rife. As well as such occasional travellers, there were people and carts going to and from the regular weekly markets and the occasional fairs, and livestock, some being driven long distances. The roads were busy with travellers, generally strung out along them but concentrating in the towns and at the wayside inns.

In their descriptions visitors to London gave the impression that it was a densely built-up city. That was true; by the end of the fifteenth century its population was roughly 50,000, within a national figure of 2.6 million. Dominic Mancini, in the mid-1480s, wrote that its 'dwelling houses are built above workshops and belong to diverse sorts of craftsmen'.[10] Mario Savorgnano, a Venetian, was in London in 1531 and he thought that the houses 'are in very great number, but ugly, and half the materials of wood, nor are the streets wide', and according to the Venetian envoy in the early 1550s, Giacomo Soranzo, London 'has a dense population'.[11] Most houses were timber-framed, with lath and plaster infilling and perhaps an outer covering of plaster; brick was in use and the chimneys were of stone. Other cities and towns attracted less attention. Visitors tended to stop at Canterbury on their way from the coast to London and to visit Oxford and Cambridge. But they generally did not reach the other large provincial cities, such as Bristol, Norwich, York, Newcastle and Exeter. Building practices were not static and an indication of change in materials was provided by John Leland, the king's topographer, who wrote in the 1540s that at Northampton 'all the old building of the town was of stone, the new is of timber'. He passed judgement on the places which he visited, such as Poole, where he found that the town was 'much increased with fair building'; he described Chester as 'chiefly one street of very mean building in length' and the cathedral as being 'of a very mean building'. He was more pleased with Exeter: 'There be divers fair streets in Exeter, but the high street ... is the fairest.' At Winchester, he noticed 'a fair hospital of St John, where poor sick people be kept'.[12] But such general impressions of places by travellers passing through them did not give an indication of the environmental issues and remedial work being undertaken to correct them.

As urban populations began to grow at an accelerating rate in the early and mid-sixteenth century, so the infilling of the centres of towns brought problems. Building in open spaces such as yards at the rear of the buildings facing the streets was often for workshops, adding to air pollution and reducing the flow of air through the built-up area. So did the addition or rebuilding of upper storeys, narrowing the gap between buildings across a street. By the 1560s the practice of jettying out the upper storeys of buildings had so irritated the city councillors at Exeter that they imposed an order fixing the dimensions of such projections and ruling that no one could build forward without the 'view and assent' of the mayor, aldermen and chamberlain. In 1563 a house owner was instructed to demolish such a jetty because it exceeded the stipulated allowance for such 'oversailing'.[13] Shoddy and insubstantial building was also likely to be a feature of urban infilling. At Worcester, an order was made in 1466 and repeated in 1496 and 1584 that there should not be any wooden chimneys or thatched roofs in the city, and the aldermen in Coventry were required by an order of 1517 to ensure that there were no wooden chimneys or thatched buildings in their ward.[14] Both in general and in detail the conditions which were thought to be conducive to disease were addressed by local administration in the cities and towns, although they could not be comprehensive with their controls.

The royal palaces could incorporate features such as windows orientated away from the moist airs. Fire destroyed the palace at Sheen in 1499 and it was rebuilt by Henry VII, who renamed it Richmond. Fire also swept through the residential buildings of Westminster Palace, in 1512, and they were not rebuilt. But Henry VIII 'builded new his place called Baynyscastell [Barnard's Castle] in London, and repaired his place at Greenwich with much new building there and in diverse places'.[15] The king and queen also had use of the royal apartments in the Tower, which were overhauled in time for the coronation of Anne Boleyn on 1 June 1533. The king had married her the previous January, having at long last achieved his objective of annulling his marriage to Katherine of Aragon. A new room was created as the queen's great chamber, which had 'a great carrall window', and new windows installed elsewhere in the buildings included a set of three in the king's dining chamber that consisted of a broad one seven feet wide flanked by two narrower ones.

Those royal buildings were augmented by Bridewell Palace, built by Henry VIII close to the Thames within the City in 1515-23, and in the second part of his reign, he greatly developed the buildings of the former York Place, the London residence of the archbishops of York, which he acquired in 1529 and made the principal royal palace in London and Westminster. The choice of the site of Bridewell flew in the face of current thinking, as the ground on which it had been built was marshy and it adjoined the River Fleet. It was scarcely ever used as a royal palace, although Henry VIII's illegitimate son Henry Fitzroy was lodged there from 1525. The French ambassador, Jean de Dinteville, lived in the palace intermittently from 1531 to 1539. Other envoys who were lodged there were the Imperial ambassador François van der Delft, from 1545 to 1550, and in 1553 Antoine de Noailles, the French ambassador. In 1553 Edward VI granted the palace to the City of London as a workhouse for the poor and vagrant populace.

Whitehall Palace had been enlarged by Thomas Wolsey before it was taken by the king. Wolsey rose under Henry VIII to be the most powerful man in the country after the king. He was appointed Archbishop of York in 1514 and Chancellor in 1515, was created a cardinal in 1516 and from 1518 was appointed successively bishop of Bath and Wells, Durham and Winchester. In the summer of 1515, Sebastian Giustinian wrote that Wolsey 'really seems to have the management of the whole kingdom'.[16] To provide space for his extra buildings he enlarged the site by acquiring neighbouring properties. The palace included state rooms and reception chambers, residential apartments, a new chapel, erected in 1528, and a long gallery. Wolsey's pre-eminent role in government, as well as the church, gave the palace a special significance as a centre for those wishing to transact official or legal business. His household consisted of roughly 500 people and was especially grand, as befitted a figure who was not only so senior in the church's hierarchy that he aspired to be elected Pope, but had a role in state affairs which required him to entertain statesmen from across much of Europe. As George Cavendish, his gentlemen-usher, wrote: 'Thus in great honour, triumph, and glory, he reigned a long season'.[17]

Wolsey fell from power in 1529 after having failed to secure an annulment of the king's marriage to Katherine, and he died in 1530. Without a London palace since the fire in Westminster Palace, Henry VIII adapted York Place. He further enlarged the site by acquisitions and reclaiming land along the riverfront, and by new building and improvements he made Whitehall the principal palace of the English crown. Land on the west side of King Street was acquired and used for recreation, with a tiltyard, tennis courts and a cockpit. It was connected to the main part of the palace by two gatehouses that spanned the street. Although the later Tudor monarchs did little to improve the palace, it certainly impressed visitors, not for any overall form or architectural distinction, which indeed it lacked, but for its interiors. In 1600 Baron Waldstein wrote that it 'fills one with wonder, not so much because of its great size as because of the magnificence of its bed chambers and living rooms which are furnished with the most gorgeous splendour'.[18]

No royal palace in or near the metropolis could be secure from infection because of the numbers who lived, worked and attended there. The court was divided into two: the household was the larger section, responsible for providing all aspects of the administration, provision and maintenance of the court, including meals, accommodation, furnishing, even transport, while the chamber consisted of those engaged in the process of government, who typically were members of the aristocracy and gentry. There was, too, the queen's chamber, with the ladies of the court. The numbers circulating around the court were swelled by those who supplied it with provisions and goods, as well as a nonstop string of lawyers and petitioners visiting their patrons to obtain support for a legal case or hoping for a position or pension. The need for security added to the numbers. Henry VII was the first English king to appoint a body of retainers to act as guards, 'to the number of about two hundred ... these he incorporated in his household so that they should never leave his side'.[19] The court numbered about 1,500 over the winter and perhaps a half of that during the summer, when the monarch made his progresses through the provinces. The size of the court would cause concern, if only because of the quantity of waste to be disposed of, which was human, animal and vegetable. Rotting garbage was thought to create the fetid atmosphere in which venomous atoms harbouring diseases could thrive. To minimise the risk of infection, the numbers with the monarch were reduced. Some courtiers moved away, for their own safety, returning to their estates, and others could be discouraged. But the numbers required to keep the king in his accustomed state were still relatively large, although the case for separation in clear air did not have to be made. The process of person-to-person infection was quite unknown, but the danger of 'miasma' was a part of Galenic medical theory and avoiding foul smells and keeping in 'clean' air was common cultural behaviour.

One way of reducing those following the monarch was for him to travel to his smaller properties. Henry VIII eventually had more palaces and houses than any other Tudor monarch, many acquired in the second half of his reign, after the fall of Wolsey and the dissolution of the monasteries. As well as York Place and Hampton Court Palace, the archbishopric of York had handed over to the king other houses, including The More and Tyttenhanger, in Hertfordshire, both of which were relatively small and were liked by Henry. Indeed, The More was described as 'a goodly house and a place fit to receive the Count Palatine' and, as with his other houses, the king enlarged and decorated it, installing his arms and insignia among the ornamentations. Among the royal houses around the capital was the new one of Nonsuch in Surrey, begun by Henry in 1538, which was a hunting lodge with limited accommodation rather than a palace.[20] Many of the smaller houses were large enough only for the king and his servants, members of the Privy Chamber and his inner circle of courtiers. They could be regulated to ensure that no one admitted showed any symptoms of sickness. Even so, the gentlemen who went ahead to plan the king's progress had to be assured that there neither was nor had been any disease in the area. If that were discovered to be the case, then an alternative had to be found; no chances could be taken. Of course, if no royal house were available the king could avail himself of someone else's if it were more suitable. In 1526 it was explained to Wolsey that 'the King intended to have stopped at Stanstyd and Southwike; but as the parish in which the former stands is infected with plague, he will go to Warblington, a house of my lady of Salisbury, two miles distant. Thence he will go to Porchester Castle, and next day to Winchester'.[21] If a member of the king's travelling party showed the symptoms of a malady, he or she was left behind when he moved on. Rules issued for the management of Edward IV's court had included the stipulation that there should be 'no perilous sick man to lodge in this court, but to avoid [leave] within three days'. Enforcement of that order was one of the duties of the king's physician, or 'Doctor of Physick'. He also advised the king on his diet and prescribed his medicines. Subordinate to the physician was a 'yeoman apothecary' who not only provided medicines but also fumigated the king's clothes to prevent infection.[22]

After Henry VIII came to the throne in 1509, Thomas Linacre was appointed as royal physician. He was becoming a leading figure in medicine in England and was a member of the humanist circle around Erasmus. He was both popular and 'skilled' in his profession, as a practical physician as well as a theoretician. Erasmus consulted him for practical advice when he was afflicted by a ringing in the ears and, on another occasion, was suffering from a fever. Linacre studied in Italy from 1487 until 1499; his reputation rested chiefly on his translations of Galen's works from Greek into Latin. He was instrumental in the establishment of the Royal College of Physicians in 1518 and was its first president. Its royal charter granted the college powers to license and oversee medical practice, and to prevent unlicensed practitioners. The college consisted of only 20 fellows, which indicates the size of the profession in early sixteenth-century England. Although its responsibilities included providing advice and information respecting plague in London, it was not set up to deal with emergencies such as the appearance of a new disease; contagion was not part of classical medical theory and the college's membership followed Galen's teachings. The physicians were the elite of the medical professions and could charge high fees from their well-off patients. The citizens who were unable to meet their charges relied instead on the medicines sold by the apothecaries, or mixtures concocted by 'wise women' with practical experience. Those who contracted the sweating sickness and were treated by such 'false leeches' stood little chance of survival, according to Forestier, who condemned their medicines and other remedies as worthless, but he thought that some victims, who received an approved medicine 'and if he purge himself before', could recover.[23]

The foundation of the college had been preceded in 1511-12 by the first parliamentary enactment about medical matters, which set out to regulate the profession. The preambles to Acts of Parliament were commonly used to describe in no uncertain terms how bad things were in the field that was being regulated and thereby justify the changes that the legislation was making. This was no exception, for the preamble declared that 'the science and cunning of physic and surgery (to the perfect knowledge whereof be requisite both great learning and ripe experience) is daily within this realm exercised by a great multitude of ignorant persons, of whom the greater part have no manner of insight in the same, nor in any other kind of learning'. Some were illiterate, the preamble alleged, and because of the lack of regulation such 'common artificers, as smiths, weavers, and women, boldly and accustomably take upon them great cures, and things of great difficulty, in the which they partly use sorcery and witchcraft, partly apply such medicines unto the disease as be very noxious, and nothing meet therefore, to the high displeasure of God, great infamy to the faculty, and grievous hurt, damage, and destruction of many of the King's liege people, especially of them that cannot discern the cunning from the uncunning'. The Act therefore ordered that no one within London or seven miles of it could act as a physician or surgeon unless licensed by the Bishop of London or the Dean of St Paul's, acting with the advice of four physicians, or for surgery 'other expert persons in that faculty'.[24] Such regulation should have assured patients of the competence of the doctors treating them, but by limiting the numbers of practitioners in that way it also reduced the numbers of people who could receive treatment, which already were very restricted.

Constrained by the intellectual limitations of the Galenic system, the physicians' faulty diagnostic skills and limited ability to prescribe effective treatments laid them open to belittling comments by humourists. They included Erasmus, the most caustic and effective satirist of the century. In his book *In Praise of Folly* he observed that 'the more ignorant, reckless, and thoughtless a doctor is the higher his reputation soars even amongst powerful princes. In fact medicine as it is practised now by so many is really only one aspect of flattery'.[25] Erasmus's views on the drawbacks of medicine as then practised were influenced by his family's experiences. His parents died of plague, his mother when she was caring for him while he was at school. When he was in the third form 'the plague, which was raging there, carried off his mother, leaving her son now in his thirteenth year. As the plague grew daily more and more severe, the whole house in which he lived was deserted, and he returned to his native place'. Plague touched many families and made many children orphans and, not surprisingly, he was very wary of diseases thereafter.[26]

John Caius's advice was to 'seek you out a good physician, and known to have skill ... and fly the unlearned as a pestilence in a commonwealth. As simple women, carpenters, pewterers, brasiers, soapball-sellers, poulters, hostellers, painters, apothecaries (otherwise then for their drugs)'. Some had come to England claiming to have served 'Emperors, kings and queens' and to have cures for 'all diseases, yea uncurable, with one or two drinks ... of great and high prices, as though they were made of the sun, moon, or stars, by blessings and blowings, hypocritical prayings, and foolish smokings of shirts smocks and kerchiefs, with such others their phantasies, and mockeries, meaning nothing else but to abuse your light belief, and scorn you behind your backs with their medicines (so filthy, that I am ashamed to name them) for your single wit and simple belief, in trusting the most, which you know not at all, and understand least.' That such a stern warning against those who took money from the gullible with rough-and-ready treatments was thought necessary by Caius in the middle of the century suggests that the problems remained, even after the earlier Henrician attempts to regulate the medical profession.[27]

Despite access to the best medical practitioners, the king and his close courtiers found safety in moving away from risks. When they felt particularly threatened the size of the group with the king was greatly reduced. Among the reasons for a progress by a small number were that he was able to move quickly and to settle a good distance from London, to deter visits and control activity. Edward IV's court regulations had provided for the movement of 'a less household than the … great sum' which had been allowed for, and nine smaller houses were listed for him to choose from.[28] In July 1516 Giustinian reported to his masters at Venice that the king had gone 'in the country' with Wolsey and Tunstall, and they were about 60 miles from London. He also suspected that 'an individual' had also gone there, said to be an ambassador from the Emperor who was trying to steal a march on his fellow diplomats by gaining direct access to the king. That made the point that although the king wished to conceal himself away from the court and the city, business still had to be conducted.[29]

Advanced warning of the presence of plague was available, with information on its presence, advance or decline accessible because of trade connections and diplomatic movements, which generated mutual exchanges of information on the presence of the disease. Those who could leave a threatened community and had somewhere to go went there and remained until the danger had passed. That was a widespread practice from the onset of the Black Death in the fourteenth century and, although those who left later attracted criticism for having neglected their fellow citizens, there was no disputing the fact that it was a sure way to survive. Yet, if an outbreak of a disease had not reached epidemic proportions, there was an argument for staying in a city. Sir Brian Tuke's wife had been dangerously ill and even, as Tuke told Wolsey, 'once or twice in danger of her life'. However, she had survived: 'being at London [she] had speedier remedy than she can have in a village', because the medical establishment was there.[30] There was a much shorter timespan for news of the indigenous disease of the sweat, because of the speed with which it spread and the swiftness with which it acted. Plague moved steadily and gave time for quarantine arrangements to be put in place, but protecting the king against the faster-moving sweat required extra vigilance.

Astrologers had continued to foretell onsets of the plague long after the Black Death, indeed throughout the long period of the second pandemic. So long as they were vague about when the outbreaks would occur they could not be wrong, for one would happen eventually. And they received a hearing. Even a rationalist such as Erasmus was willing to listen to those predictions. In March 1518 when he was planning a journey from Louvain to Basel he wrote to a friend that 'The astrologers say there will be such a pestilence this year that only men of upright life will survive, which means very few. Look after yourself'. Despite this joke, Erasmus took the predictions seriously, partly because he was apprehensive of a journey through Germany, which 'besides her long history of robberies is now exposed to the plague'.[31]

Daniel Defoe's *A Journal of the Plague Year* was published in 1722. A work of fiction, it tells the story of the Great Plague of 1665 drawing on sources from the time, but in many respects describes the responses to epidemic diseases which would have applied to the previous two centuries or more. Defoe was critical of the astrologers' influence at plague times, complaining that they 'added stories of the conjunctions of planets in a malignant manner, and with a mischievous influence' and 'if the poor people asked these mock astrologers, whether there would be a plague, or no? they all agreed in the general to answer, *Yes*, for that kept up their trade'. They did indeed find that there was a great interest in their predictions. According to Defoe:

> The terrors and apprehensions of the people, led them into a thousand weak, foolish, and wicked things, which, they wanted not a sort of people really wicked, to encourage them to; and this was running about to fortune-tellers, cunning-men, and astrologers to know their fortune, or, as it is vulgarly expressed, to have their fortunes told them, their nativities calculated, and the like; and this folly, presently made the town swarm with a wicked generation of pretenders to magic, to the black art, as they called it, and I know not what; Nay, to a thousand worse dealings with the devil, than they were really guilty of; and this trade grew so open, and so generally practised, that it became common to have signs and inscriptions set up at doors; Here lives a fortune-teller; here lives an astrologer; here you may have your nativity calculated, and the like.[32]

Plague and the sweat were constantly on the minds of those who perused reports of the presence of disease to assess the level of danger, and of those who feared it but did not have the means of ascertaining the truth. Anxiety rose and fell according to the seasons of the year, for the months when plague threatened were known; but in 1485 that feature of the sweat was yet to be established. With no overseas outbreaks to provide examples and an early warning, the sweat posed a formidable challenge to those whose responsibility it was to know about such things.

Chapter Four

The Sweat in Henry VII's Reign

Londoners who witnessed the expansion of the deadly contagion which affected their city from late September 1485 must have been aware that this was a new disease. Nothing they had experienced so far in their lives resembled it, nor had the speed and deadliness of this hitherto unknown malady. It is impossible to know what the reaction of members of a society would be to a disaster of that kind, but it is possible that some members, at least, may have hoped that this was one of the occasional diseases that struck London and that if they sat tight it would go away. That was not to be the case because the disease lingered intermittently for a hundred years.

The outbreak in London began on or shortly before 21 September; the mayor died on the 23rd and his successor succumbed on the 28th. In all, six aldermen died and by implication, roughly a quarter of Londoners perished in the epidemic. It is likely, however, that their duties exposed them to a higher risk of contracting the virus than most of the citizens and they were not a representative group, so that is an overestimate. Margaret, wife of Mayor Sir Thomas Hill, one of its victims, survived the epidemic and lived until 1501. The French physician Thomas Forestier put the number of dead from the disease in London at 15,000, a figure which may be taken to be speculative, given the absence of any form of numerical recording. But the parish clergy and officers would have been aware of the falling numbers at church services and those taking the sacrament, which gave them some general idea of the loss of parishioners. Forestier's figure probably is not far from the estimate of one-quarter of the population and supports the estimate based on the number of aldermen who had died; which, based on modern estimations of a population of 50,000 by the end of the fifteenth century, suggests a death toll in the range of 10,000 to 12,000. Although numerical precision, even approximation, was impossible in a society which did not think in such terms, Forestier's number does indicate that contemporaries were aware that the number of deaths was unusually high.

The death toll from the disease was concentrated within a few weeks, for the sickness had subsided by late October, when the king returned to London. According to the *Great Chronicle of London*, it was around the Feast of Saints Simon and Jude, on 28 October, that the 'aforementioned sickness declined, by God's forbearance and by the good and moderate care of such patients as were then afflicted'. It had lasted just over five weeks, during which, according to the *Great Chronicle* 'much people' died; the chronicler John Harding mentioned 'the great death of many a thousand men', which may refer to England and not only to London.[1]

When the outbreak began the king left London and went to Guildford in Surrey. He dared not go too far from the city, for the new monarchy was barely established and if he left a power vacuum it could be vulnerable. He therefore moved closer to London at Sheen, on the Thames (now Richmond). Anne of Bohemia, Richard II's queen, had died there of plague in 1394 and the king had then demolished the buildings. New ones were erected by Henry V in 1414, with the addition of a Carthusian monastery, and the manor served as Henry VII's refuge during the sickness.[2] As it subsided he returned to the capital and the coronation took place in Westminster Abbey on 30 October, after the customary procession through the city. He would not have gone back before the disease had subsided.

Forestier included anecdotes to stress how swiftly the virus killed its victims. He wrote that 'We saw two priests standing together and speaking together, and we saw both of them die suddenly...we see the wife of a tailor taken and suddenly died. Another young man walking by the street fell down suddenly. Also another gentleman riding out of the city died. Also many others the which were long to rehearse [recount] we have known that have died suddenly'. These were dramatic and possibly exaggerated cases, designed to show the social range of the victims (two priests, a gentleman, a tailor's wife) and that a young man could be a casualty of the epidemic. Forestier again mentioned the age range of those who were killed in his dedication of his work to Henry VII:

> When that thy highness and thy great power is vexed and troubled with divers sickness, and thy lordships and almost the middle part of thy realm with the venomous fever of pestilence, and, by the reason of that, young and old and of all manner of ages, with divers wailings and sadness they are stricken: therefore, excellent and noble prince, we are moved with every love and duty, and not for no lucre neither covetousness, to ordain a short governing against this foresaid fever.[3]

Forestier was keen to inform as many people as possible of the nature of the disease and so wrote in English, not in Latin, the language of medicine, or in his native French. And he chose to circulate the tract in manuscript; the skill of printing with moveable type was relatively new in England and either he could not interest a printer in the material or felt that copying by hand would produce copies as quickly. Perhaps unwisely, he mentioned the current chatter that the dead at Bosworth had been left on the field unburied, which was contrary to accepted practices and reflected badly on Henry Tudor's conduct and his new regime. That would have been most unwelcome to the monarchy and perhaps for that reason Forestier was arrested and imprisoned in the Tower. He was connected to the Plantagenet regime, for in January 1485 Richard III had granted him a lifetime's annuity. The copies of his tract, which were in English, were confiscated, apparently quite efficiently because only one copy has survived. That is not entirely surprising, for even in the populous city of London those who were literate would have been known and the copies could have been traced among them. An indication of this comes from an incident in the spring of 1516 with the pasting of a notice on the door of St Paul's and another one on Lady Barking's door criticising the king and council by claiming that foreigners obtained 'much money' from the king, and bought wool to the undoing of Englishmen. The official response to the bill was 'great displeasure' and an attempt to identify the perpetrators by taking a sample of the handwriting of everyone in the City who was literate. That was to be done by assigning a member of the king's council to every ward, who was to co-operate with the alderman of the ward and identify those who were literate, taking an example of their handwriting to the guildhall. Clearly, the Council was confident that the number of those within London who were literate was small enough for them to be identified and that the sample of handwriting which they produced was manageable enough for that of the guilty person to be matched with the offending notice. The incident indicates that the aldermen were expected to know their own wards in detail, and explains the seizure of the copies of Forestier's tract. His conduct while in detention may have been defiant, for when Henry VII granted him a general pardon in January 1488 it was 'for all escapes and evasions out of the Tower of London or elsewhere, and remissions of forfeiture of all lands and goods'. Forestier then left England and returned to Rouen, where he expanded and published his tract in 1490, in Latin; only four copies of that version have survived.

His focus was on London, where an alderman was the senior official representing each of the 24 wards into which the City was divided for administrative purposes; the Court of Aldermen was the city's ruling body, providing the agenda for the much larger Common Council, the legislative body. In 1485, 33 men served as aldermen because of the unusual number of deaths. By the loss of so many of its leaders in such a short space of time, the City lost their experience of administering its affairs; Sir William Stokker had been an alderman since 1470, Sir Thomas Hill since 1473, Richard Rawson since 1476, John Stokker since 1479 and Thomas Northland since 1481, and Thomas Breteyn was serving as Sheriff when he died. Their livery companies similarly suffered losses among their senior members. The disruption caused by the outbreak is suggested by the lack of any wills enrolled in the Court of Hustings for that year.[4] But the City gained two major benefactions from the aldermen's deaths. In his will Sir Thomas directed that within five years of his death the City should 'provide the means and ways to have the water at Paddington to be conveyed by pipes of lead from thence unto the great conduit of the City of London and to other places of the same city if it shall seem to them necessary so to do' and a conduit should be made at Gracechurch Street, to receive and hold some of that water. According to his directions 'one fair conduit of sweet water castellated with crest and vent' was built there by his executors, who paid the whole cost out of his estate.[5] From Rawson's bequests the building at St Mary Spital where the aldermen sat for the annual sermon, which was one of the major events in fifteenth-century London, was purpose-built in 1488 by his executors and those of his wife Isabel. He also bequeathed £20 towards 'the bringing home' of a new water pipe to the conduits in London and gifts to the leper hospitals around the city.[6] Those bequests probably would have come to the City in due course, but the timing was because of the deaths of the two men in the epidemic of sweating sickness.

The disease seems to have diminished after causing the epidemic in London, rather than spreading outwards from the city along the internal trade routes and by sea to the coastal ports. References to it are sporadic, such as one from Norfolk on 23 September, which mentions an unspecified 'sickness' which may have been the sweat, and the abbot of Crowland Abbey on the edge of the Fens died of it on 14 November. It was also present in western and southern England by October, and it may have lingered in the Midlands, through which Tudor's army had passed during the summer and where the outbreak was said to have 'lasted but a month or six weeks'. After the Battle of Bosworth Henry VII 'gradually lessened his army ... dismissing those who had been summoned from the northern borders to take part in the expedition'.[7] If the disease had been rife in the army, it might be assumed that the returning soldiers transmitted it as they dispersed. But no substantial mortality has been traced in any region: the record of wills in Hertfordshire shows an increase in deaths in the autumn of 1485, but not a spectacular one, while the counties of East Anglia experienced no such rise. Individual cases may not have been enough to spread the disease to the point where it became a general outbreak. It may be that the virus steadily lost its virulence during the year and that it did indeed increase and cause suffering among those infected, but they recovered and, without a marked rise in deaths and a corresponding number of wills, it left no trace in the record. This runs counter to the impression given by chroniclers that it infected much of the country in a deadly epidemic: a record from the West Country refers to a 'sudden sickness in all places of England'. Or it may be that the change in the weather during the autumn brought the epidemic to a halt, as the virus did not spread readily in damp and cool weather, which indicates that it was not an influenza-type disease. It did not recur as a significant killer in the following spring and so 1486 was not a year when the sweating sickness made an impact outside individual localities.[8] What is clear is that, as in so many other examples, the disease which accompanied a military campaign or followed it caused far more deaths than did the fighting.

The subsequent years down to the late 1490s did not see an epidemic of plague, which was an unusually long gap between outbreaks in the fifteenth century. When the next epidemic did strike, in 1498, it then continued until the following decade and affected many places. The epidemic was a severe one, described as 'a great pestilence throughout all England', during which 'men died in many places very sore; but especially and most of all in the city of London, where died in that year thirty thousand'.[9] It is likely that, notwithstanding that estimate, 10,000 died in the city during the outbreak, or roughly 20 per cent of the population. Norwich suffered in 1500 and again in 1503-4, York in 1501 and 1505-6, Worcester in 1502 and Chester in 1506. The disease responsible for the high mortality was plague; the sweat was not mentioned.

A number of the king's senior counsellors died in the years around the turn of the century and the royal family lost the king and queen's youngest son, Edmund, who had been born in February 1499 and died in June 1500. Two of their sons remained: Arthur, Prince of Wales, who was born on 19 September 1486, and Henry, who was born on 28 June 1491. After a long period of diplomatic negotiations, Arthur was married on 14 November 1501 to Katherine, daughter of the Spanish monarchs Ferdinand and Isabella. This was quite a diplomatic coup for England's relatively new dynasty, which was still not altogether secure from the claims of pretenders to the throne. The most dangerous of them was Perkin Warbeck, who claimed to be the Duke of York, Edward IV's younger son, who was not disposed of until he was executed in 1499 at Tyburn. His co-conspirator, the young Earl of Warwick, the last of the Plantagenet male line, was beheaded on Tower Hill.

In December, the month after their wedding, the young royal couple travelled to Ludlow, where Arthur established his court. A Council for Wales and the Marches had been established by the king in 1490 and Arthur was its titular head. Edward IV had made a similar arrangement, creating the Council in 1472 for his son Edward, Prince of Wales, and adding to its authority. Edward could have been a titular head of the Council only, but he was sent to Ludlow as a boy, presumably to learn, or at least observe, the way in which royal authority was maintained in that region. Henry VII copied that arrangement and despatched Arthur there after his marriage. John Leland described Ludlow as 'set upon a hill; so that a man coming to it any way conscendeth it. It is well walled, and by estimation it is about a mile in compass'. As a market town with a thriving wool trade and, with the presence of the Council, an administrative centre, it was prosperous enough to have developed suburbs outside its gates. The castle was close to but not within the town and the retinues of the senior figures there did not need to interact with the citizens, although suppliers came and went.[10] The residential apartments were in ranges within the inner bailey, which was relatively small and entered through one gateway. Few visitors would have penetrated so far and most would have conducted their business in the much larger outer bailey, which contained the castle's chapel of St Peter. The castle had been one of the possessions of the Langley family, earls of Cambridge and dukes of York, and so became a royal castle on the accession of Edward IV in 1461. In contemporary terms it did not have an unhealthy setting, but did have a fluctuating population, drawing in eager suitors and petitioners as well as those who were required there to serve the Council. Arthur had long-standing links with the region and in March 1493 he was appointed as the king's Justice in Shropshire, Herefordshire and Gloucestershire and in the Marches of Wales. Thereafter he was an occasional visitor to the town, with the Council.[11]

Arthur never left Ludlow after his arrival with Katherine, dying there on 2 April 1502. Both the king and queen were grief-stricken at the loss of their eldest son, and his death had a major political significance, for in a short space the king's male heirs had been reduced from three boys to just one, Henry. The queen became pregnant again shortly after Arthur's death and gave birth to a baby girl, named Catherine, on 2 February 1503. She died in infancy and the queen also died, nine days after giving birth; the king did not remarry. Arthur, meanwhile, had been buried in Worcester Cathedral, where King John was buried, and a decorated chantry chapel was built to house his tomb; work on the chapel was begun in 1504. Katherine remained bedridden for a time, perhaps stricken by the disease which had killed her husband. At least one member of his household also died, for among the 'graves of men of fame in the church' noticed by Leland was that of 'Cokkis, a gentleman servitor to Prince Arthur'.[12]

Katherine's parents, Ferdinand and Isabella of Spain, wrote on 12 May to their ambassador telling him that she was 'suffering' and should be moved as soon as possible 'from the unhealthy place where she now is', and in another letter mentioned that at that place 'the situation is unhealthy'. They followed that up with the instruction that the princess should be allowed the revenues from her dowry in full, that she and her advisers must not borrow any money and that 'all the gold, silver, jewels, &c. of the Princess' must be kept with the greatest care and that 'Not the smallest portion of them ought to be sold.' Her household was not to be changed until the arrival of their special ambassador. Information soon reached them that the king had already moved her from 'the unhealthy situation where she was staying, and that she has come to a place nearer London'.[13] Although reassured on that point, their anxieties relating to finances, status and diplomacy remained. Sir Francis Bacon later wrote that astrologers had been consulted about the match between

Arthur and Katherine, adding that 'it is not good to fetch fortunes from the stars'.[14]

The Spanish monarchs were not the only anxious parents in the aftermath of Prince Arthur's death; Henry VII had invested his political hopes in his eldest son, perhaps at the expense of instructing Henry for a political role, and he now had to take extra care with his sole male heir. Henry was carefully protected, at least that is implied by a remark made by the Spanish diplomat Don Gutierre Gómez de Fuensalida that he was kept under minute supervision, more suited to a girl, and 'so subjected that he does not speak a word except in response to what the King asks him'.[15] Although created Prince of Wales, Henry was not sent to Ludlow, and was largely brought up at the royal palace at Eltham, south-east of London and close enough to it for the young prince to be in touch with the court. Ludlow had been rather remote.

Prince Henry's reaction to his brother's death was not recorded, but it must have shocked him profoundly, especially as it was shortly followed by the deaths of his mother and infant sister. Those sad events emphasised the fragility of existence and the future of the dynasty, responsibility for which would fall to him. Although the hazards of life were obvious to all and royalty could not be shielded from them entirely, perhaps the depredations of disease could be tackled; certainly, the precautions taken by some foreign governments suggested that was the case. How far Henry's thinking came to move along such lines is unknown, nor is the extent to which his brother's death made an impact on his awareness of his own mortality (he was just ten years old at the time), but in adult life, he displayed an undue nervousness about his health which may partly have stemmed from Arthur's premature demise.

Contemporaries reacted more strongly to the consequences of Prince Arthur's death than to its cause. He had been ill for two months after his arrival at Ludlow and on 27 March, which was Easter Day, his condition worsened significantly and there 'grew and increased upon his body the most pitiful disease and sickness, that with so sore and great violence, had battled and driven [itself] in[to] the singular parts of him inward'. Eventually 'that cruel and fervent enemy of nature, the deadly corruption, did utterly vanquish and overcome the pure and friendful blood, without all manner of physical help and remedy'. That is the only description of Arthur's ailment and it provides little guidance for a historical diagnosis, yet antiquarian writers and modern historians have ventured to suggest that the sweating sickness was responsible. That does not fit the description, for the sweat acted swiftly and its victims did not linger, it was active during the summer not during the spring, and 1502 was not a year when it is known to have caused deaths elsewhere. Katherine's illness took a long time to shake off and almost certainly was the same malady which had killed Arthur. From the description of the disorder that afflicted the royal couple, we may be sure that it was a disease other than the sweat that was responsible. Suggestions have included bubonic plague, which was unlikely because of the length of the illness and the absence of a mention of the distinctive, and well-known, symptoms, and tuberculosis, which was improbable because the disease develops very slowly and would have been recognised and commented on sooner than was the case.[16] Evidence of deaths in Herefordshire shows a peak around the time of Arthur's death, with an earlier peak in November 1502 which was especially marked in the deaneries of Ludlow and Leominster. Arthur could well have succumbed to an infectious disease that made an impact regionally, but not further afield, and which is not identifiable from the information provided by the single description.[17]

According to Caius, the sweating sickness 'came again' in 1506, the 22nd year of the reign. John Stow wrote that in that year 'the sweating sickness ... now assailed them again, howbeit, by the remedy found at the beginning of it [the reign] nothing the like number died thereof, now this second time, as died the first'. If he was correct, then it may be that the outbreak was less virulent than that 20 years earlier, or the population had developed some resistance to the strain of the virus; no effective treatment had been concocted.[18] Scattered references indicate that the disease struck quite widely across England and in places made the same devastating swift impact as it had done in London at its first onset. A history of Norwich mentions the outbreak, but rather dismissively: 'In 1506, was the second sweating sickness, but not so raging as the first'.[19] But at Chester it killed 91 householders in three days in 1506–7, equating to perhaps 500 people in all.[20] At Creake Abbey in Norfolk the 'infectious or epidemical disease' that killed several of the canons may have been the sweat; the abbot died on 12 December 1506 and as insufficient canons remained to elect a successor the abbey was effectively dissolved and reverted to the crown.[21]

The chronicler Bernard André dated the second outbreak to 1508, and that was accepted by the nineteenth-century historian Charles Creighton. André was a French Augustinian friar who had attached himself to Henry VII's court after 1485 and thereafter dedicated his poetry and other works to the king. A blind scholar, he was given the responsibility for Prince Arthur's education, from 1496-1500. André wrote that in July 1508 some members of the Lord Treasurer's household contracted the disease and died 'and everywhere in this city [London] there die not a few'. In the following month, prayers were offered in St Paul's for deliverance from the disease. The pattern was established which was to become common in the later outbreaks, of the king and his immediate entourage moving quickly from place to place to avoid the malady. He went to Hatfield on 9 August to visit his mother, then moved to Wanstead but there some of his household 'sweated', so he went to Barking and then to other places; by then it was about the middle of the month. He avoided Greenwich and Eltham because members of the establishment in both royal palaces 'had sweated'. Three members of the king's privy chamber were infected, which was an ominous development because it showed that the measures in place to evade the disease were ineffective. Perhaps even more alarming were the deaths of three of the prince's privy chamber. It must have seemed that the disease could not be avoided, for the two courts were well separated, with the king and his entourage at Richmond and Hanworth, to the west of London, and the prince's household centred upon Eltham, to the south-east of the city. Messengers probably would have passed between the two but would surely have been aware enough to stop short of entering the buildings or coming close to members of the households. That endangered the future of the dynasty, with both the king and his heir under threat despite the care taken to isolate them. The impression, reinforced by André, was that the sickness 'then raged in all places' and that there was no escaping it. In a development which prefigured later actions, an order was issued on 17 August that no one from London should go near the court and no one from the court should go to the city. Physicians and apothecaries were exempt from the controls, but there were few of them. By the end of August the epidemic had ceased; the king and the prince both survived, but the disease had claimed the lives of some high-profile figures. Among those who died in the epidemic were Geoffrey Simeon, formerly Dean of the Chapel Royal and then Dean of Chichester, and John Lord Greystoke, who died in August. Greystoke was a pupil of the Lord Privy Seal, Richard Foxe, Bishop of Winchester, who survived the disease and went on to found Corpus Christi College, Oxford.[22] It seems that there were outbreaks of the sweat in both 1506 and 1508, widely dispersed around the country and varying in intensity.

Contemporaries would not have been surprised to hear of the evasive actions that Henry took. There were several premature deaths among young members of the royal and ducal families of western Europe around the turn of the century, including those of Arthur and Edmund Tudor. They wrecked dynastic plans and brought children and inexperienced adolescents to the throne. The future ruler of Spain, Austria, the Netherlands and much of the Americas, and future Holy Roman Emperor as Charles V, was brought up by his aunt Margaret of Austria at her court in Mechelen, north of Brussels. She was a careful custodian of her nephew and other Habsburg children in her care, writing on one occasion that 'even the slightest illness in people of such importance causes concern'.[23]

Henry VII had been in poor health before his summer progress in 1508 and he died on 21 April 1509. He had suffered from a recurrent disease that, like that which had claimed Prince Arthur, is now unidentifiable. Also like the prince, the king lingered on in growing pain for at least three weeks after he had realised that he was dying. In his will he acknowledged the need to make provision for the poor who were sick or in poverty, stating that the works 'most profitable, due and necessary, for the salvation of man's soul' were 'visiting the sick, ministering meat and drink and clothing to the needy, lodging of the miserable poor, and burying of the dead bodies of christian people' and that the remedy was 'common hospitals, wherein if they be duly kept, the said needy poor people be lodged, visited in their sicknesses, refreshed with meat and drink, and if need be with clothes, and also buried if they fortune to die within the same'. Yet he admitted that 'there be few or none such common hospitals within this our realm, and that for lack of them, infinite number of poor needy people miserably daily die, no man putting hand of help or remedy'. He had begun the process of establishing such a hospital on the site of the Savoy Palace, near Charing Cross, for 100 poor people: 'Sick or lame, or travellers; to be furnished with lodging, food, firing and attendance'. It was dedicated to St John the Baptist and a statue of the saint was placed over the Strand gate. The buildings were completed between 1515 and 1517 and were staffed by a master, four chaplains, a matron and twelve sisters. That was on the site of the palace of John of Gaunt, one of Edward III's sons, which had been wrecked by the rioters during the Great Revolt of 1381, and not restored, so he was bringing back into use as a charitable foundation a site which in its heyday had been symbolic of royal wealth and as such had aroused the wrath of the citizens. Henry also directed that similar hospitals should be established at York and Coventry, although that was not done. He assigned the vast sum of £33,500 to complete and endow the three institutions, a measure of his commitment to the care of the sufferers and in marked contrast to his reputation, then and later, as a miserly man.[24] The need to look after the sick and poor was recognised and provision made for their maintenance in this way, but prevention and cure were still far in the future.

His son and successor Henry VIII was born after the first onset of the sweating sickness, but the next deadly one had probably subsided only about eight months before he succeeded his father, and it seems probable that the rapid evasive actions taken in 1508 made quite an impression on him. It had shown that, as well as the plague, the disease was a real threat to the monarch and his courtiers, as well as being an excruciating illness that spread both fear and death. The attempts to isolate the king taken during that epidemic included the beginning of a growing set of rules aimed at securing the monarch's safety during epidemics.

Chapter Five

A Sickly Decade

The new reign brought a sense of relief, with the accession of a young, athletic and accomplished king, who quickly became popular. He swiftly enhanced his favourable reception by ordering the arrest of his father's financial enforcers, Richard Empson and Edmund Dudley, and releasing Sir William Capel, who had been Mayor of London in 1503 and was to be again in 1510. But the young king's reign began with an epidemic, as his father's had done. Edward Hall wrote that there was 'a greate Pestilence in the town of Calais, and much people died', and a few lines later added that in 1509 'the plague was great, and reigned in divers parts of the realm'.[1] The plague was the agent responsible for the epidemic; the sweat was not mentioned.

Members of the intellectual circles in London, Oxford and Cambridge were especially hopeful that the new reign would bring patronage and encouragement. Lord Mountjoy sent a long letter to Erasmus, encouraging him to return to England, praising the new king to the skies as 'a prince whose exceptional and almost more than human talents you know so well'. He went on to wish that Erasmus could see 'how happily excited everyone is here, and how all are congratulating themselves on their prince's greatness'. He anticipated a complete change of mood: 'Heaven smiles, earth rejoices; all is milk and honey and nectar. Tight-fistedness is well and truly banished. Generosity scatters wealth with unstinting hand'.[2] In personal terms his optimism was not misplaced, for he was knighted at the king's coronation on 23 June 1509 and shortly afterwards was made Master of the Mint. That letter to Erasmus may in fact have been written by Andreas Ammonius, Mountjoy's secretary. The promise of patronage would certainly have appealed to Erasmus, but his reservations about the English environment had to be overcome. Over the next few years, he corresponded with Ammonius, who was appointed Latin Secretary to the king in July 1511 and was in Henry's entourage during the military campaign in France in 1513. Ammonius also found favour with Thomas Wolsey, who arranged his appointment as collector in England of Peter's Pence, a papal tax. He supplanted Polydore Vergil, who resented Wolsey's actions in displacing him from that post to make way for Ammonius and thereafter became a hostile critic of the great man, which was to find expression in his history of the period.

Ammonius was born in Lucca in 1476 and travelled first to Rome before arriving in England by 1506. Vergil was born near Urbino around 1470 and he, too, had a spell in Rome and then arrived in England in 1502. Both men were drawn to England by the circle of Italians around Giovanni Gigli, who was appointed Bishop of Worcester in 1497, and his nephew Silvestro Gigli, who succeeded him as bishop in 1498 and died in 1521. Ammonius did admit to Erasmus in 1511 that he regretted leaving Rome and his friends there, who had prospered, but in fact he was an integral member of the European-educated humanist circle in England that included Thomas More, John Colet, Richard Pace, William Grocyn, William Lily and Thomas Linacre.

Ammonius's correspondence with Erasmus expressed, among other things, his misgivings about living conditions in England. He told Erasmus that 'I am quite out of sympathy with this nation's dirty habits, habits with which I am already well enough acquainted, and yet my poverty will not permit me to take a lease of a house and live as I should like to live'. Accommodation was a long-standing problem for Ammonius. He was dissatisfied with his lodgings and had been told of a community of lawyers near St Paul's 'who, they say, live rather well', but he did not fancy it, to put it mildly: 'in my opinion it would be living in a sewer'. The Italian merchants in London lived together in a community and that was also recommended to him, but he had some misgivings and did not take up the offer.[3]

Despite Ammonius's reservations, Erasmus did return to England in 1511, staying in London before moving to rooms in Queens' College, Cambridge. While in London he experienced an attack of sweating sickness, which was so bad that rumours of his death reached as far as Mechelin, in the Low Countries, and Bologna, in northern Italy. On 25 August he told Ammonius that 'my health is still a little shaky as a result of that sweating sickness I told you of'. He was reluctant to return to London that autumn because of a plague outbreak there. On 5 October he asked Ammonius 'whether the plague is as bad as common report has it'. Clearly, it had not reached Cambridge. Three weeks later Ammonius told him that in London 'we have not yet come to terms with the plague' and not until early November could he report that the plague 'has almost ceased to rage'.[4] There was no possibility of mistaking the sweat for the plague, especially by such an anxious observer of diseases as Erasmus, yet 1511 was not noted as a year in which the sweat was active, or even as an epidemic year for any illness. It may be that the plague outbreak, following on from the sweat later in the summer, took attention away from the sweat and the two diseases came to be described together as a 'plague'.

In 1513 there were plague deaths in London and Cambridge, with the university closed during October. Erasmus retreated to the nearby village of Landbeach, where he gathered news of the plague's progress. He made two forays to London to collect his belongings from his lodgings, which he was reluctant to do. Eventually he steeled himself and 'in complete solitude' went there to pack his books and other possessions for collection and then 'I hurried away and never even slept in my room'. His caution was understandable, for during October plague deaths numbered 300 to 400 daily in London, two of the Venetian ambassador's servants fell victim to the disease in August and the ambassador himself left the city in fear. The servants' bed, sheets and other belongings were thrown into the Thames. Erasmus found that in London 'all were fleeing' and in Cambridge, in late October, 'Everyone is running away … in all directions.' In truth, the plague was 'very prevalent in England'.

Erasmus summarised his, and probably the current, thinking in a letter to William Gonnell, a schoolmaster in Cambridge:

> There is no reason ... for you to be much perturbed at the death of one or two people, unless the scourge begins to spread in all directions; especially when, as things are in England at present, changing one's domicile simply means changing, and not escaping from, one's danger. Avoid the contagion of a crowd as much as you can; live temperately as you are doing; and keep the members of your household from contact with crowds in the same way. Winter is upon us now; and winter commonly cures troubles of this sort.

That was written in early November.[5] Plague was described as the cause throughout that year's epidemic and there was no mention of the sweating sickness, although had it been present the advice would surely have been similar. Erasmus's optimism that the disease would disappear during the winter was misplaced; he wrote in the middle of February 1513 that it was still unsafe to go around London because of the plague. In August 1513 one of the butlers at the Inner temple died of the pestilence 'And the great plague at that time was in London, therefore everyone was discharged from commons at his pleasure'.[6]

Disease continued to disrupt the life of the city and court over the following years. In May 1514 a papal delegate visited England to make a formal presentation. That went ahead in St Paul's cathedral as planned, with the king in the procession, but the meal served at the palace, which was to be expected, did not take place. The king went to Eltham for Whitsuntide and 'because certain near the Court were dead of the great sickness, [he] kept no household save for his chapel and office of arms'.[7] The house of the Poor Clares at the Minories suffered terribly during an epidemic in 1515 when 27 nuns and some of their servants died, virtually the entire house.[8] Such a death toll was unusual in a plague epidemic and suggests that, once the disease had been identified among them, the nuns may have agreed that they should all remain within the site and not risk spreading the venom by fleeing. Or perhaps the speed with which the disease ripped through the community took its members by surprise, which suggests that the sweating sickness was the agent. An unspecified ailment struck the Earl of Shrewsbury's household in April 1516; Wolsey's advice could have been his reaction to any infectious disease: 'Counsel my lord to get him into clean air and divide his household in sundry places, and if the danger of sickness be past by the next term then to be at London'. The sickness was attributed to the 'contagious plague' and before the end of the month 'They begin to die in London, in divers places, suddenly, of fearful sickness'. The speed of death implied does suggest that the sweating sickness was the cause, although that was rather early in the year for it to be virulent enough to cause deaths.[9]

The preferential terms allowed to foreign merchants, especially those from the Low Countries, were a source of long-standing resentment in London. In 1517 that boiled over in the Evil May Day riot, which was the most serious outbreak of violence in London during the sixteenth century. May Day was a traditional holiday for London's apprentices and journeymen who were accustomed to misbehave in a way that was mild enough to be overlooked. But that year the simmering discontent as the holiday approached was more threatening than usual. Yet the actual trigger for the violence was not necessarily a major affront to the citizens. One suggestion was that the cause was an Italian who had abducted a goldsmith's wife and purloined some of his silver, and another that a servant of the French ambassador had taken two doves from a stall-holder without paying for them. They were not major incidents. Sebastian Giustinian attributed the origins of the disturbance to an inflammatory sermon by one Dr Beal at Paul's Cross during which the preacher 'commenced abusing the strangers in the town, and their mode of life and customs, alleging that they not only deprived them of their industry, and of the emoluments derivable thence, but disgraced their dwellings, taking their wives and daughters; adding much other exasperating language, persuading and exhorting them not to suffer or permit this sort of persons to inhabit their town'.[10]

Whatever the spark which ignited the smouldering resentment among the apprentices, early in the morning of May Day they 'rose up

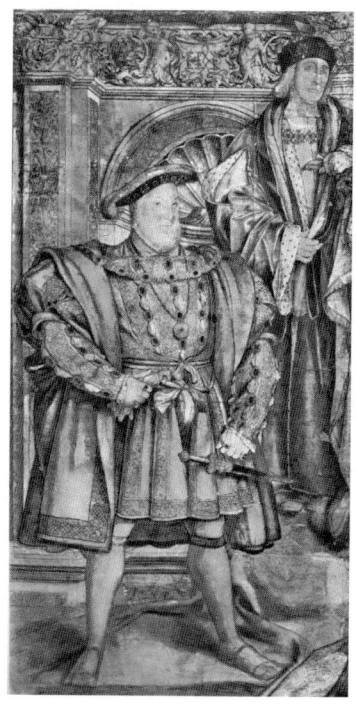

Henry VIII with his father Henry VII by Hans Holbein the Younger, 1537. This preliminary drawing was part of a design for a wall-painting in Whitehall Palace. (© *Stephen Porter*)

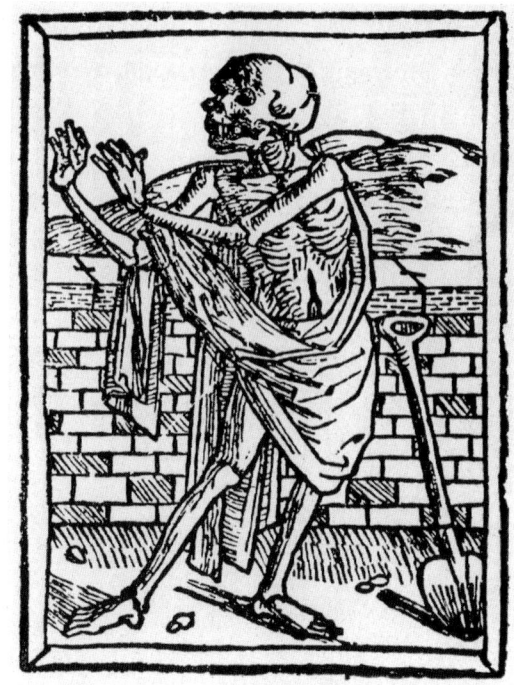

Woodcut showing Death as a gravedigger from Des Dodes Dantz, Lubeck, 1489. (© *Stephen Porter*)

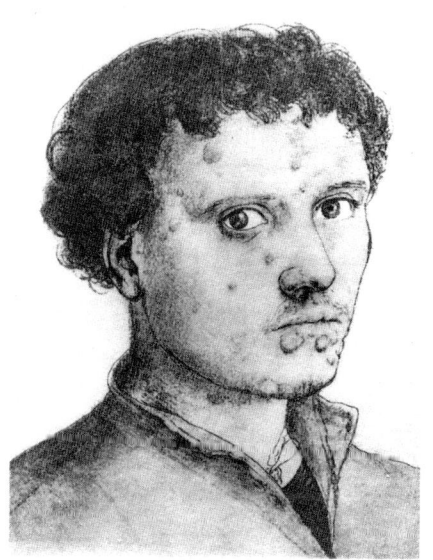

The Leper by Hans Holbein the Younger. Despite the provision of leper houses, proclamations continued to ban lepers from entering cities and mixing with the rest of the population. (© *Stephen Porter*)

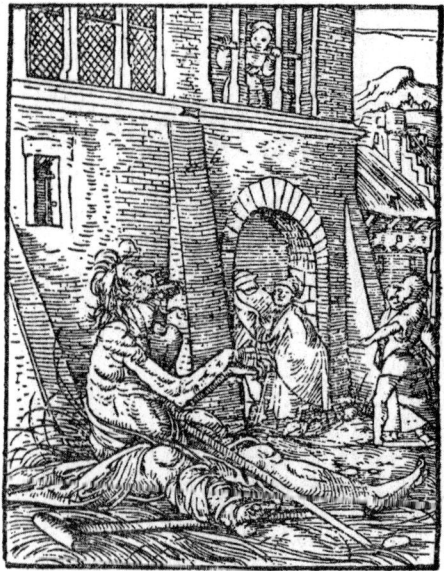

Woodcut of The Beggar by Hans Holbein the Younger. The sweating sickness threatened everyone from the king in his palace to the beggar at the rich man's gate. (© *Stephen Porter*)

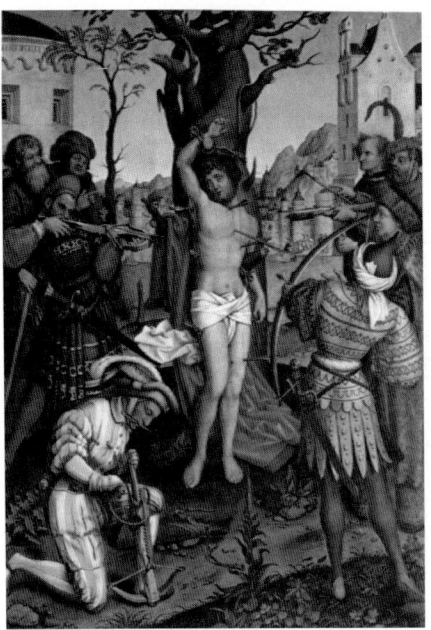 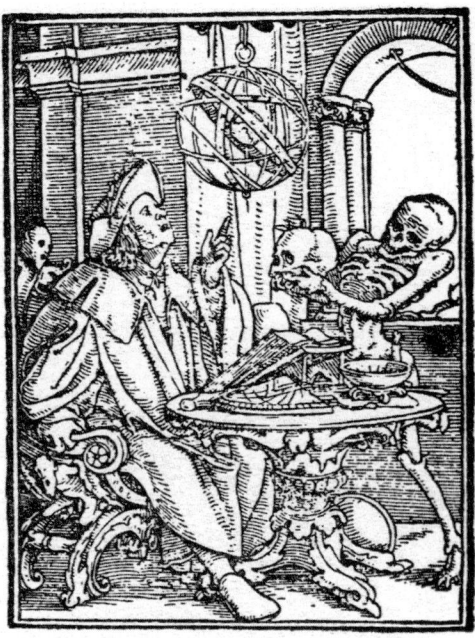

The Martyrdom of Saint Sebastian by Hans Holbein the Elder, 1516. During an epidemic, people implored the saints to safeguard them, and Saint Sebastian became associated with plague. (© *Stephen Porter*)

Woodcut from The Dance of Death by Hans Holbein the Younger. An astrologer studies a celestial globe while Death offers him a skull. Astrologers foretold outbreaks of pestilence. (© *Stephen Porter*)

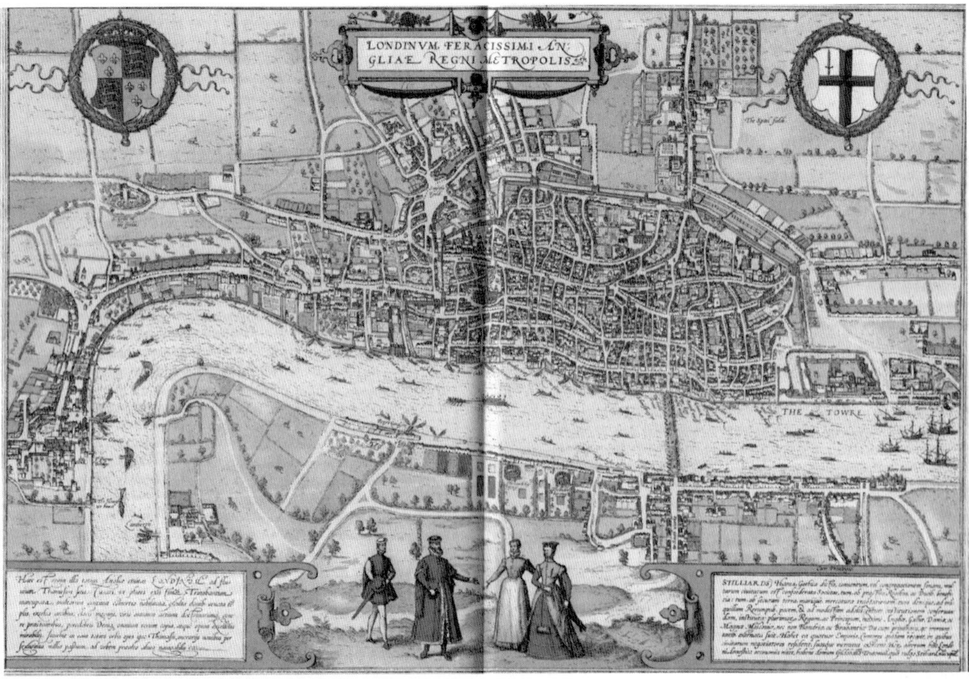

Map of London by Braun and Hogenberg, 1572. Cities and towns were not the ideal places to be when epidemics struck with some commentators blaming the inhabitants' filthy habits and lack of cleanliness for causing disease. (© *Stephen Porter*)

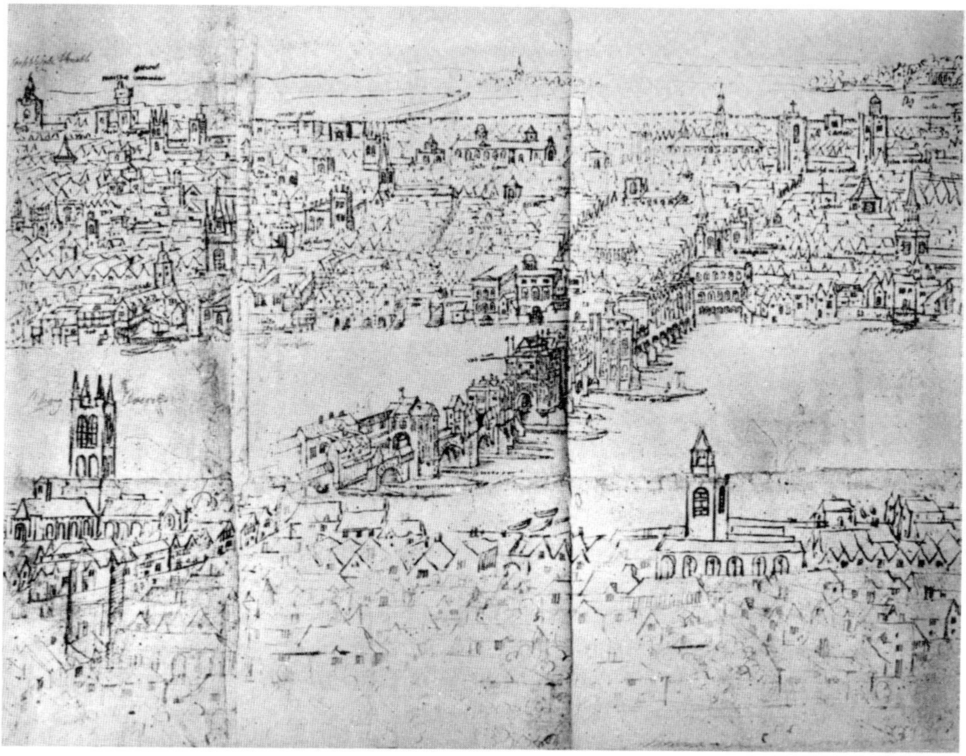

View of London from the south featuring London Bridge by Anthony van Wyngaerde, 1550. (© *Stephen Porter*)

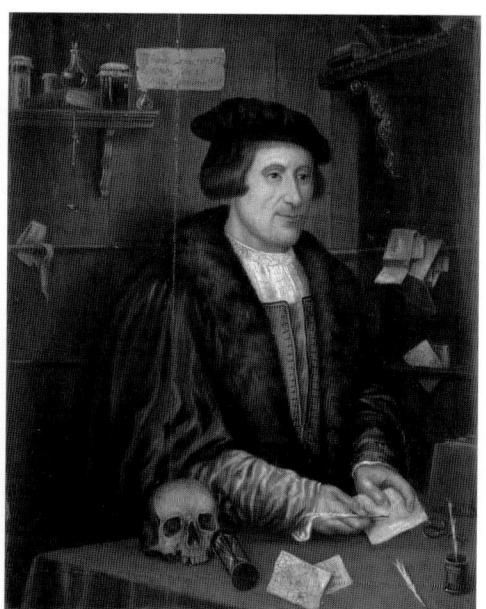

Oil painting of a man considered to be Thomas Linacre. Linacre was appointed Royal Physician when Henry VIII became king. (© *Public Domain: Wellcome Collection*)

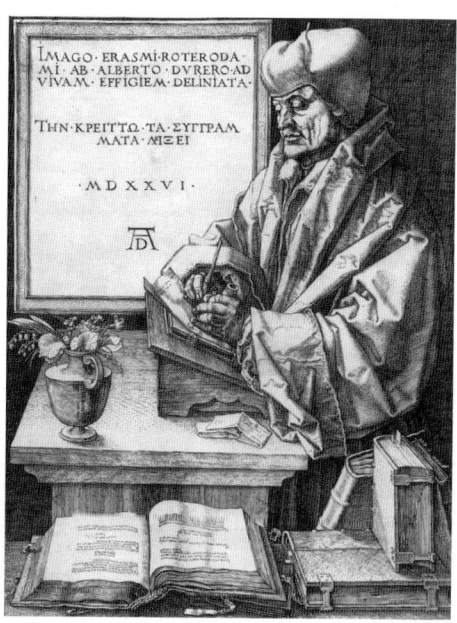

Desiderius Erasmus by Albrecht Durer. The humanist scholar Erasmus was an anxious observer of diseases as he travelled across Europe. (© *Stephen Porter*)

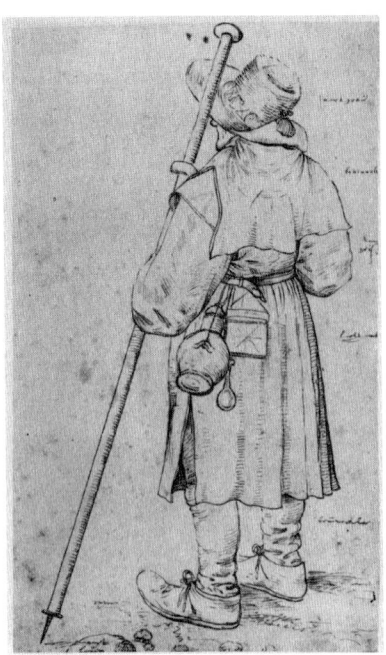

A pilgrim by Pieter Bruegel the Elder. The Church regarded the Black Death as divine punishment for sin, so when plague struck some people undertook pilgrimages to holy places. (© *Stephen Porter*)

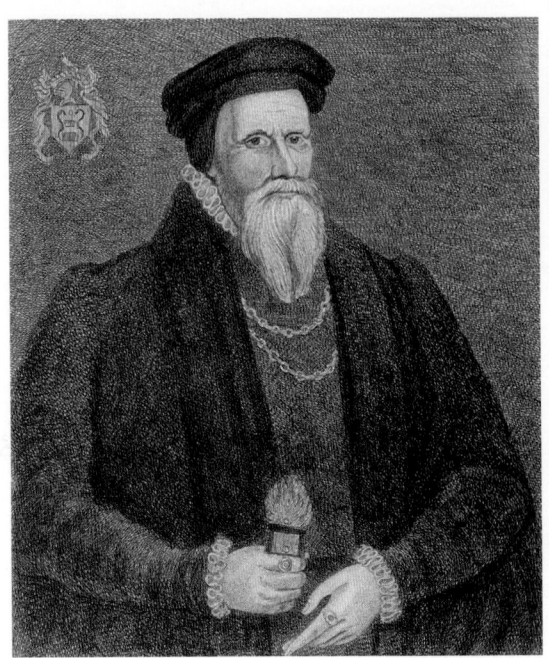

Engraving of John Caius by Charles George Lewis, 1801. The Padua trained physician Caius wrote a tract on the sweating sickness. (© *Public Domain: Wellcome Collection*)

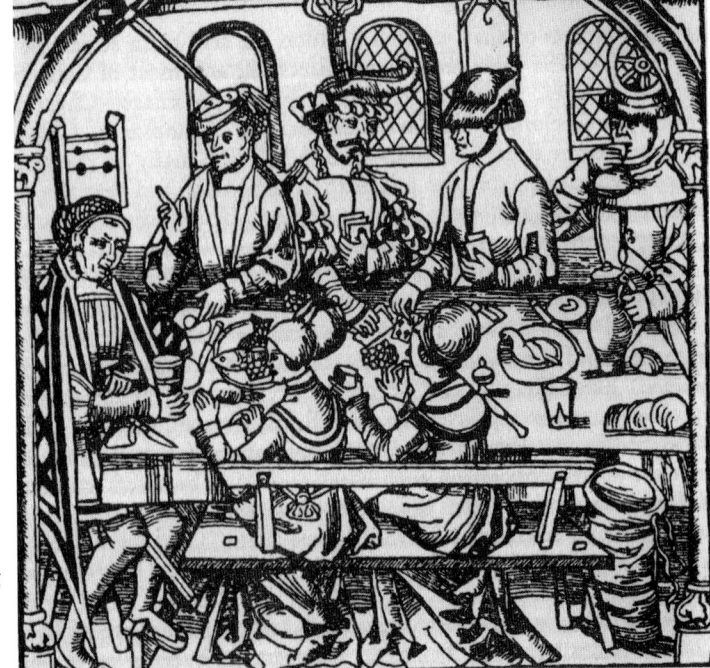

Woodcut of a Tudor tavern. The physician John Caius thought that lifestyle increased susceptibility to the sweating sickness, singling out "good ale drinkers, and Tavern haunters". (© *Stephen Porter*)

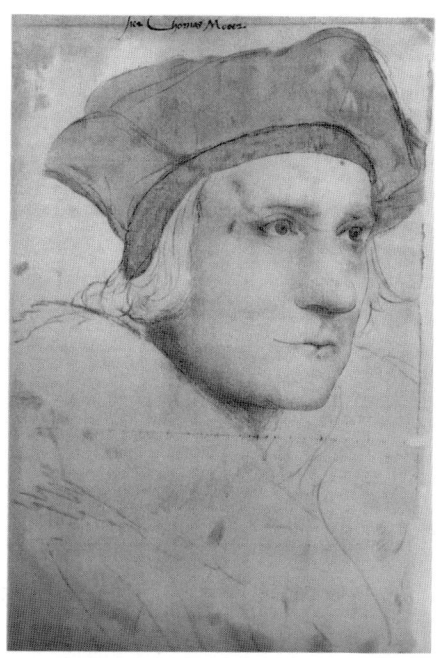 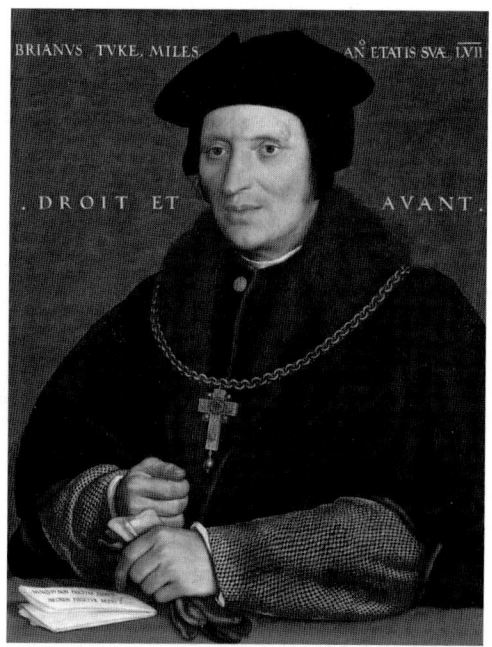

Drawing of Thomas More by Hans Holbein the Younger. Thomas More was a prominent intellectual and Chancellor of England 1529-32. He favoured the 'sweet fresh air' of the countryside, contrasting it with the oppressively closed surroundings in the city. (© *Stephen Porter*)

Portrait of Sir Brian Tuke by Hans Holbein the Younger. Tuke was appointed Treasurer of the Chamber in 1528. His wife survived the sweating sickness but was left very weak by it. (© *Public Domain: National Gallery of Art, Washington, Andrew W Mellon Collection*)

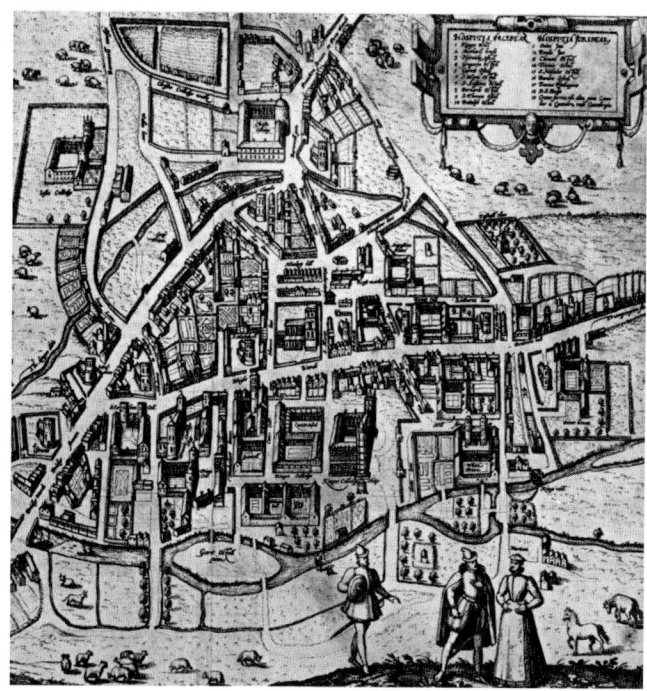

Map of Cambridge by Braun and Hogenberg, 1575. Students at Cambridge ran the risk of contracting the 'Cambridge Sweat', an almost annual occurrence which was not helped by the city's cold and damp climate. (© *Stephen Porter*)

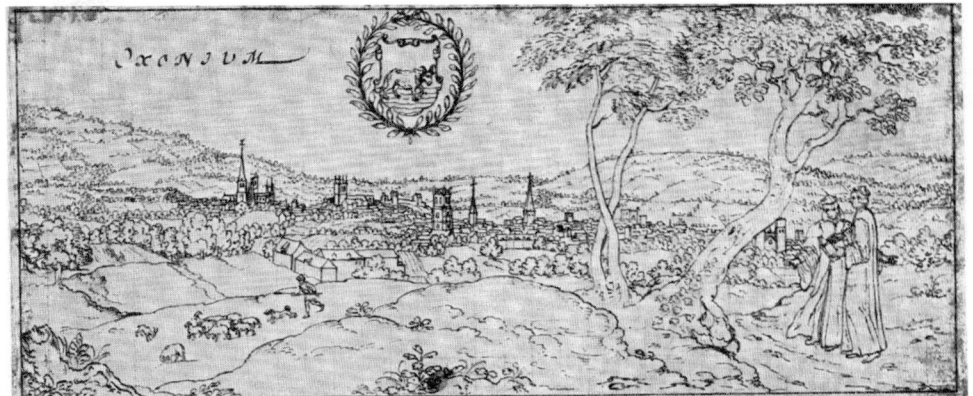

View of Oxford by Joris Hoefnagel. Oxford had a reputation for being unhealthy and in the late 15th and early 16th centuries recorded twice as many deaths as births. (© *Stephen Porter*)

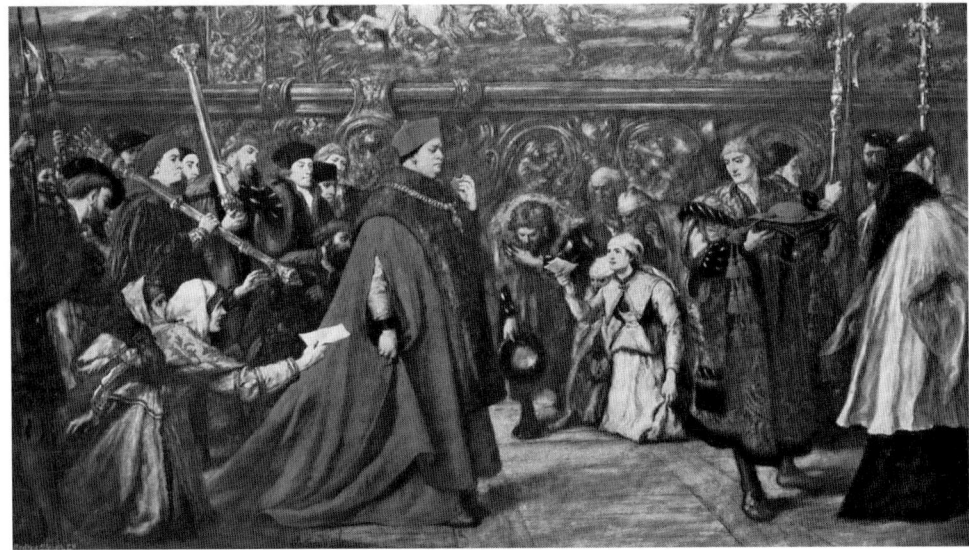

Painting of Cardinal Wolsey on his way to Westminster Hall by Sir John Gilbert. Thomas Wolsey, the King's chief minister, was in the habit of carrying 'a very fair orange', from which the inside had been taken out and replaced by 'the part of a sponge, wherein was vinegar and other confections against the pestilent airs.' (© *Stephen Porter*)

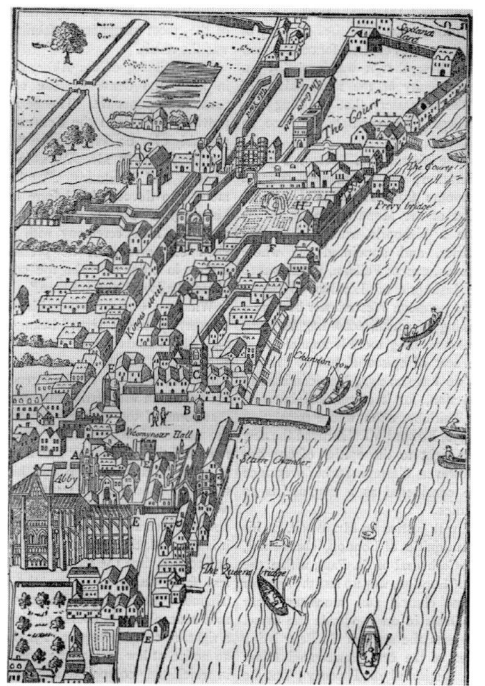

A bird's eye view of Whitehall and Westminster in the 16th century based on the Agas Map. (© *Stephen Porter*)

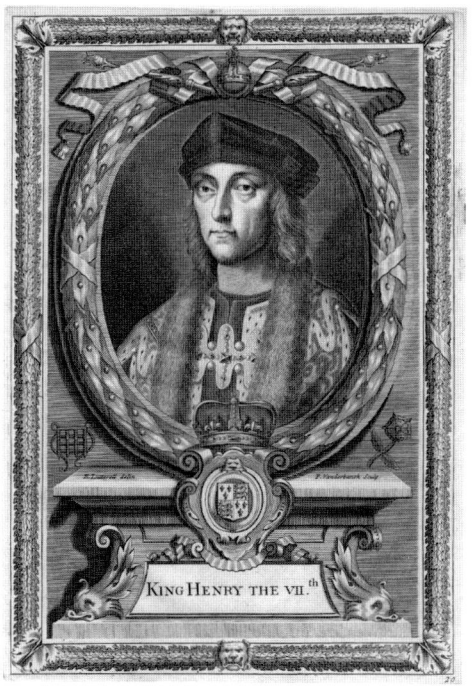

Engraving of Henry VII by Edward Luttrell. Henry VII's accession in 1485 coincided with the first appearance of the sweating sickness epidemic in England. (© *Stephen Porter*)

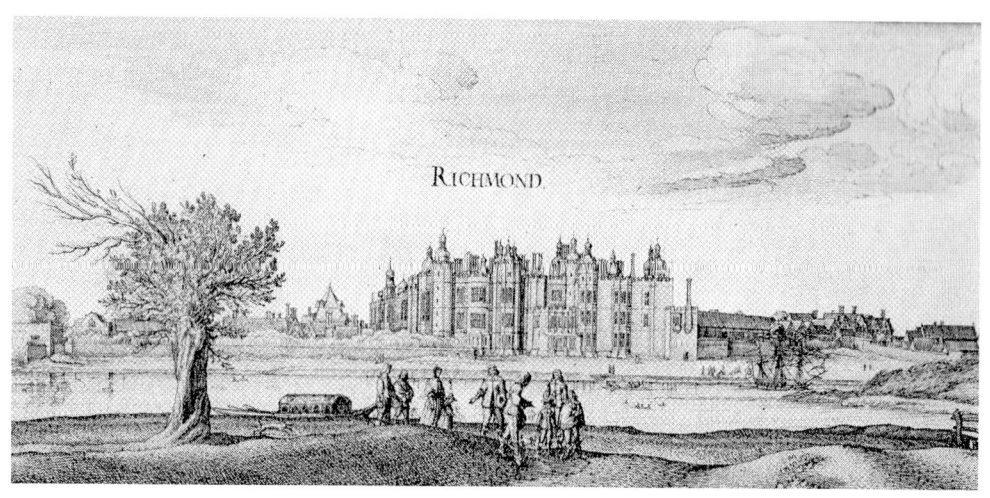

Richmond by Wencelaus Hollar, 1638. After a fire, Henry VII rebuilt the old palace at Sheen and renamed it Richmond. The King and his entourage retreated to Richmond to escape the sweating sickness. (© *Stephen Porter*)

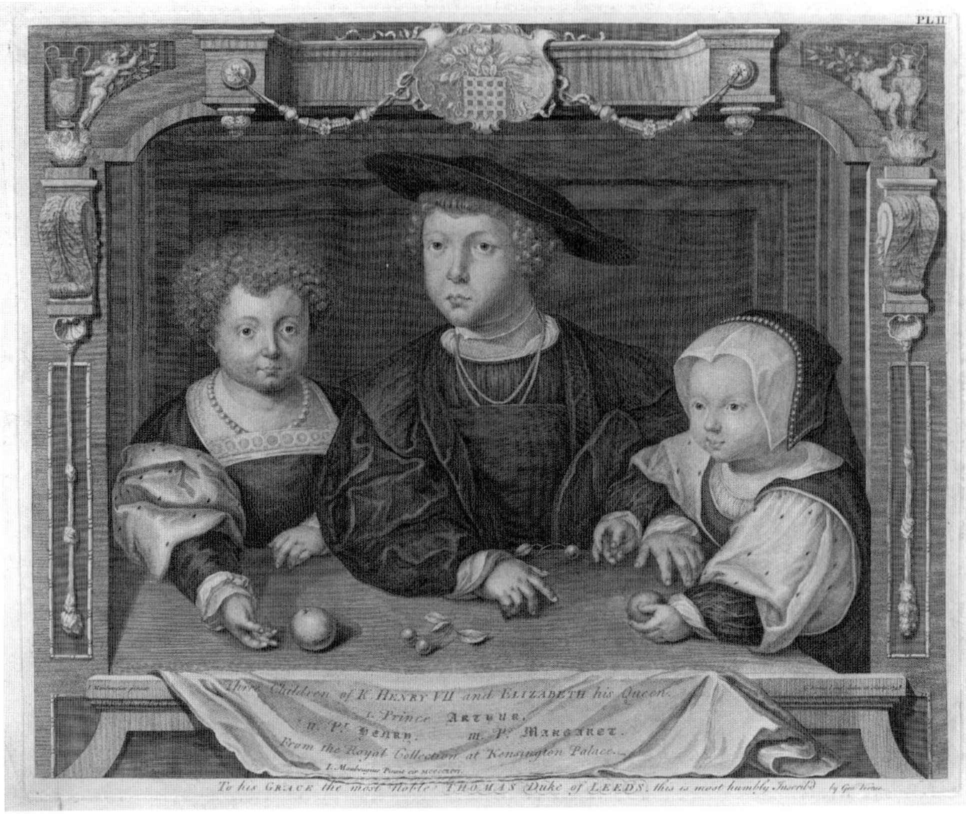

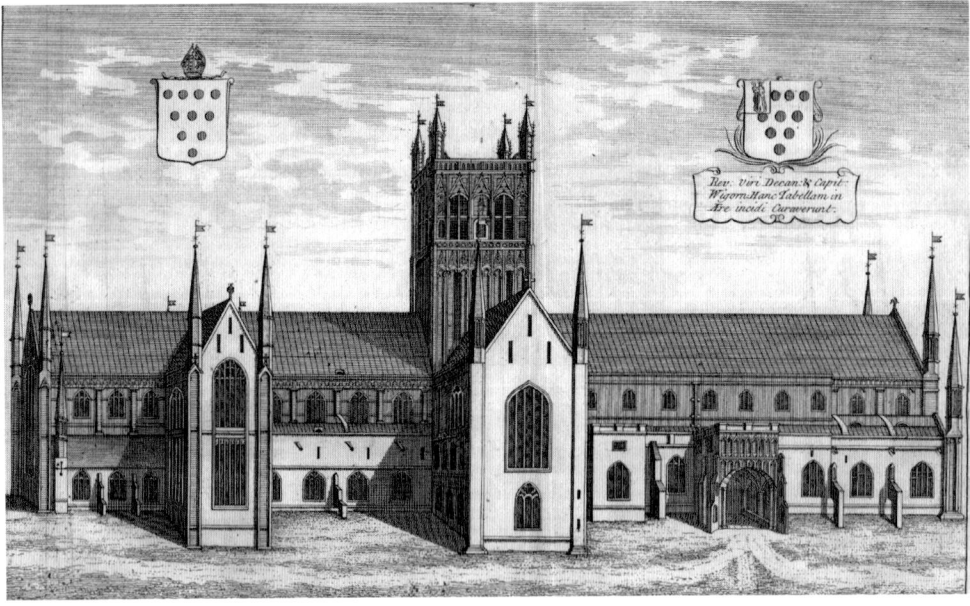

Three children of Henry VII by George Vertue. The etching shows the heir Prince Arthur flanked by his siblings Prince Henry and Princess Margaret. (© *Public Domain: Yale Center for British Art*)

Cathedral Church of St Mary at Worcester by Harris. The fifteen year old heir to the throne Prince Arthur died of an identified illness in 1502 and was buried in Worcester cathedral. (© *Stephen Porter*)

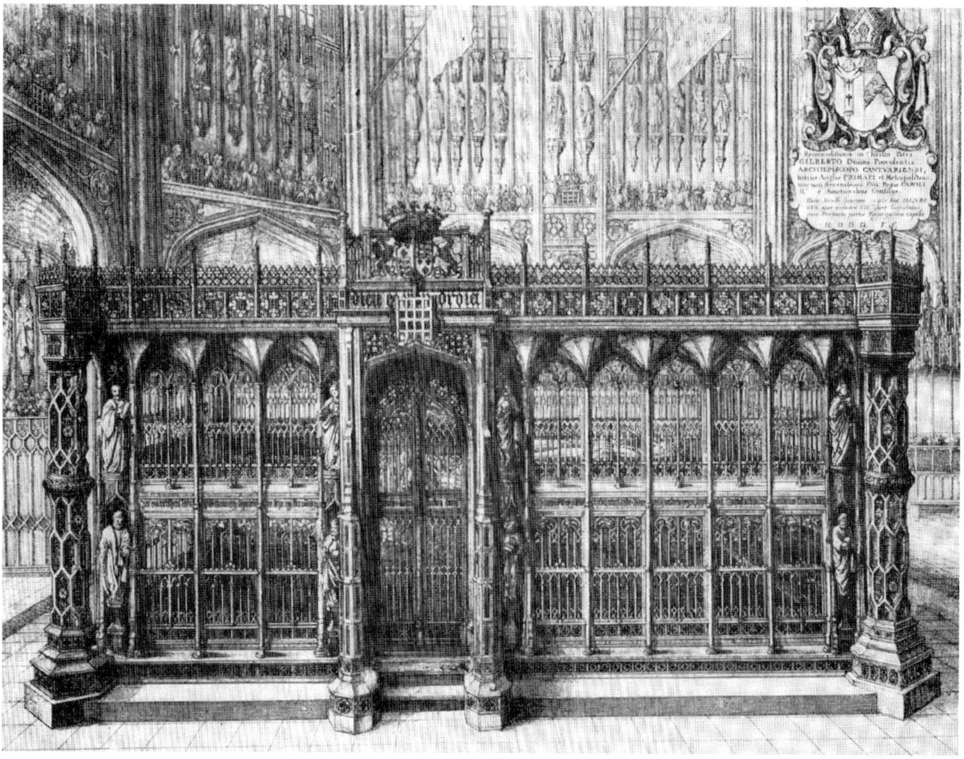

The Tomb of Henry VII in Westminster Abbey by Wenceslaus Hollar, 1665. Henry VII died in 1509 after a period of poor health. (© *Stephen Porter*)

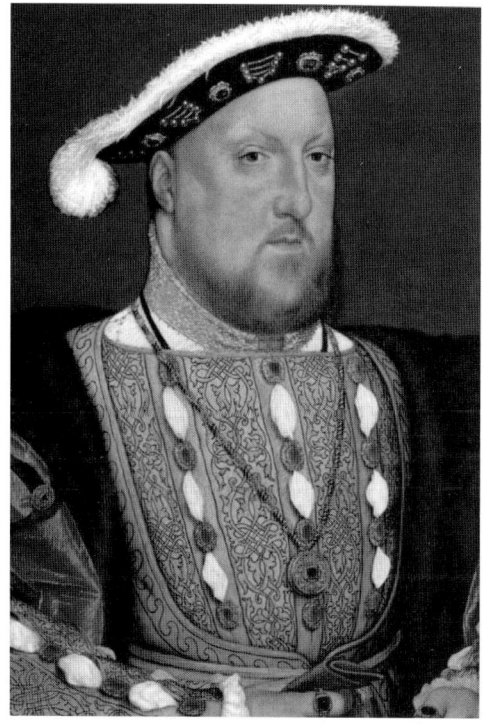

Portrait of Henry VIII by Hans Holbein the Younger, circa 1537. (© *Stephen Porter*)

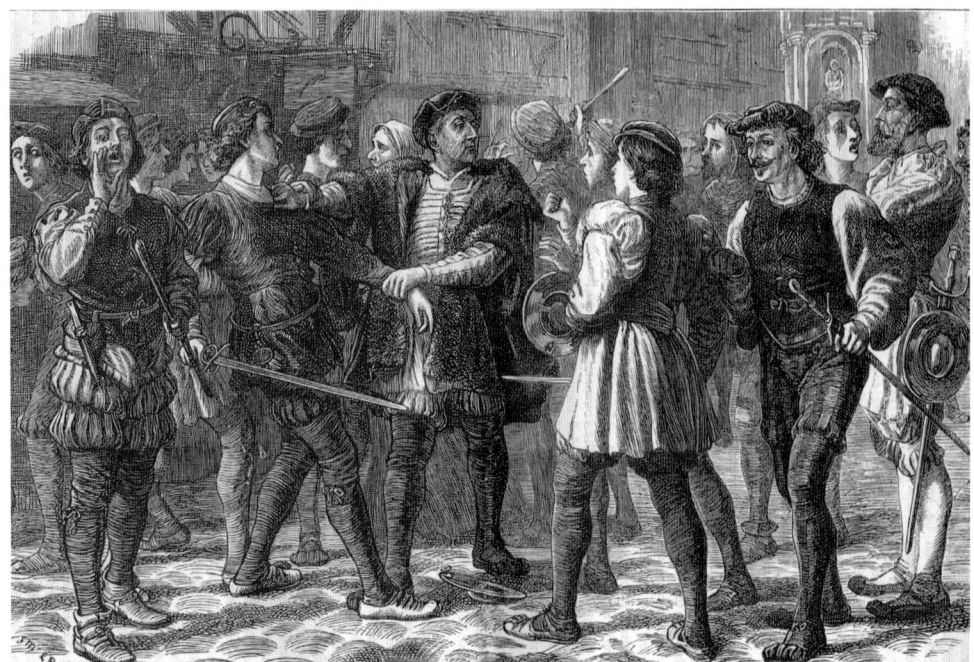

On May Day 1517 Londoners' latent hostility to the Flemish and French in the city boiled over into a riot led by the apprentices. (© *Stephen Porter*)

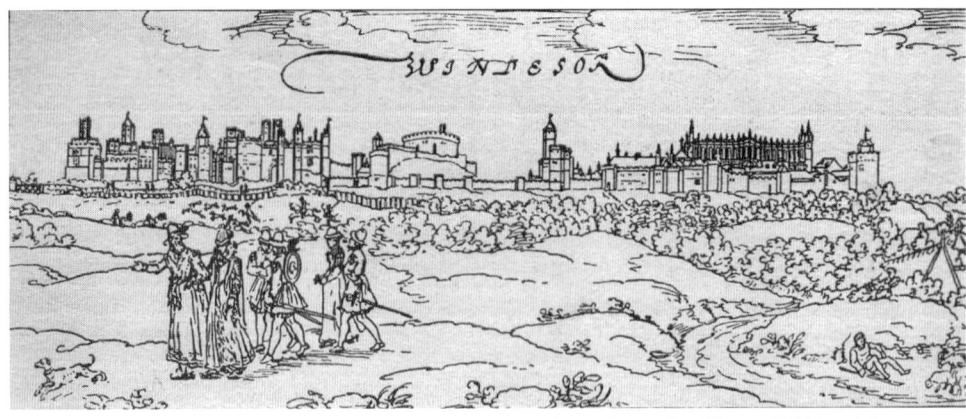

View of Windsor by Joris Hoefnagel. Windsor was one of the places that Henry VIII could retreat to when sickness threatened. (© *Stephen Porter*)

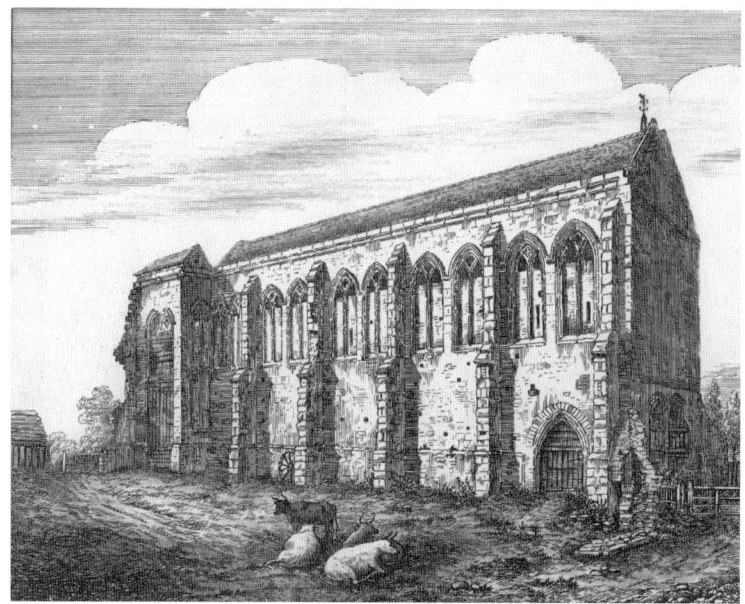

Engraving of the Hall of Eltham Palace, 1796. Henry VIII was largely brought up at the royal palace at Eltham, south-east of London. (© *Public Domain: Yale Center for British Art, Paul Mellon Collection*)

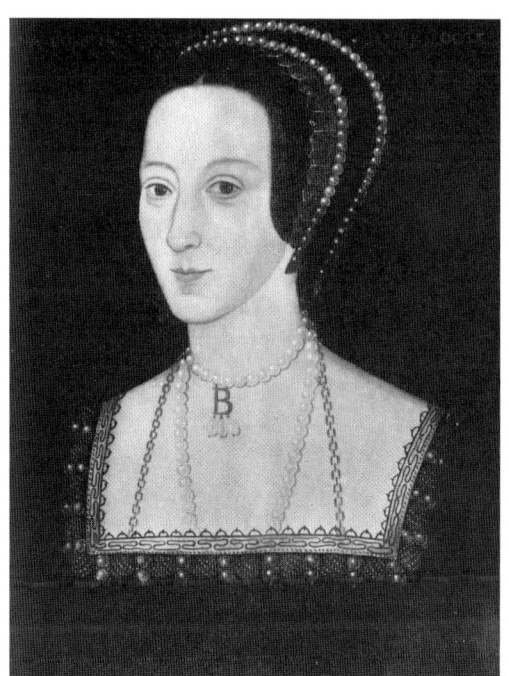

Portrait of Anne Boleyn after Hans Holbein the Younger. Both Anne and her father, Sir Thomas Boleyn, caught the sweating sickness and recovered. (© *Stephen Porter*)

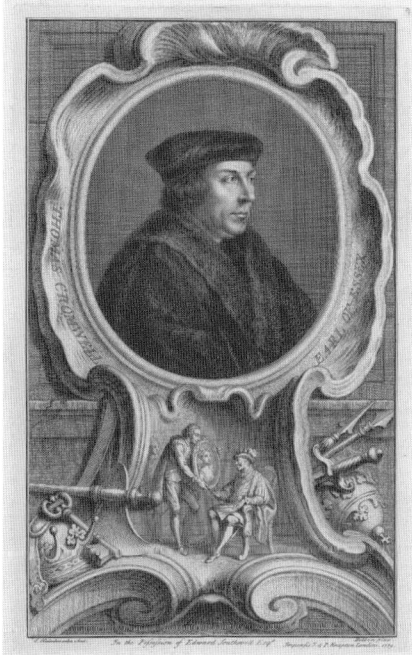

Engraving of Thomas Cromwell by Jacobus Houbraken, after Hans Holbein the Younger, 1739. Thomas Cromwell succeeded Wolsey as Henry VIII's chief minister. (© *Public Domain: Yale Center for British Art; Yale University Art Gallery Collection*)

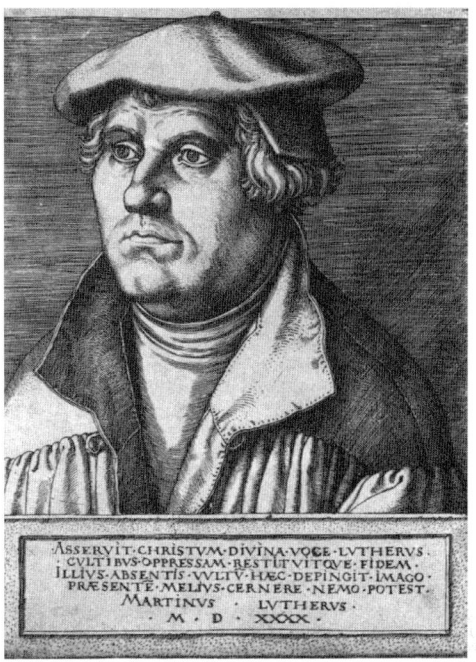

Engraving of Martin Luther by Heinrich Aldegrever, 1540. According to Luther, the discussions of the reformers at Marburg castle ended prematurely because of the threat of the sweating sickness. (© *Stephen Porter*)

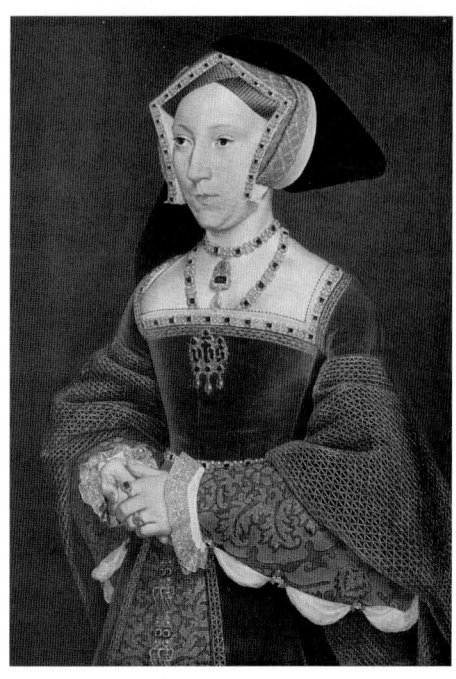

Portrait of Jane Seymour by Hans Holbein the Younger, 1536. Jane was Henry VIII's third wife but died shortly after giving birth to the future Edward VI. (© *Stephen Porter*)

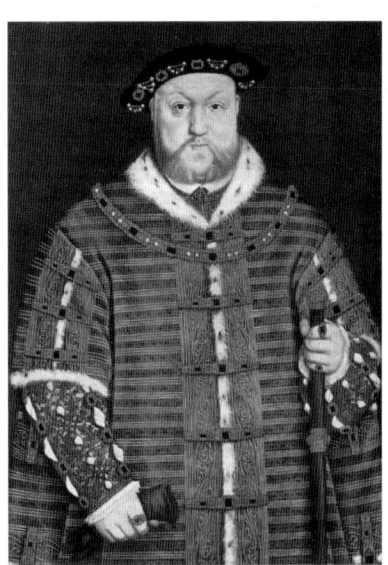

Portrait of Henry VIII by Hans Holbein the Younger, 1542. (© *Stephen Porter*)

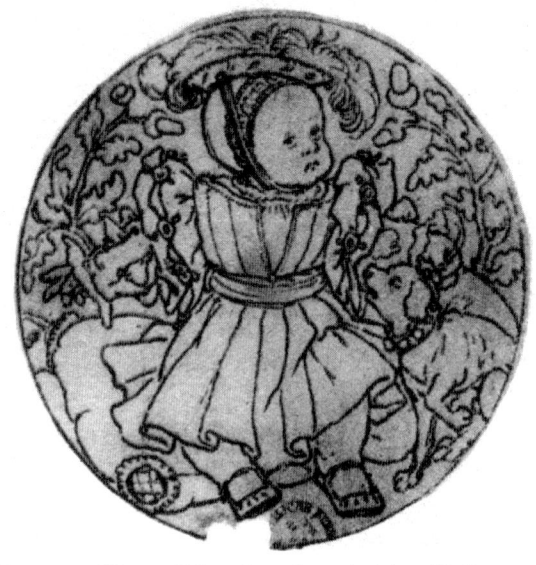

Drawing of Prince Edward aged two by Hans Holbein the Younger, circa 1539. Edward wrote that he was 'brought up [un]til he came to six years old, among the women'. (© *Stephen Porter*)

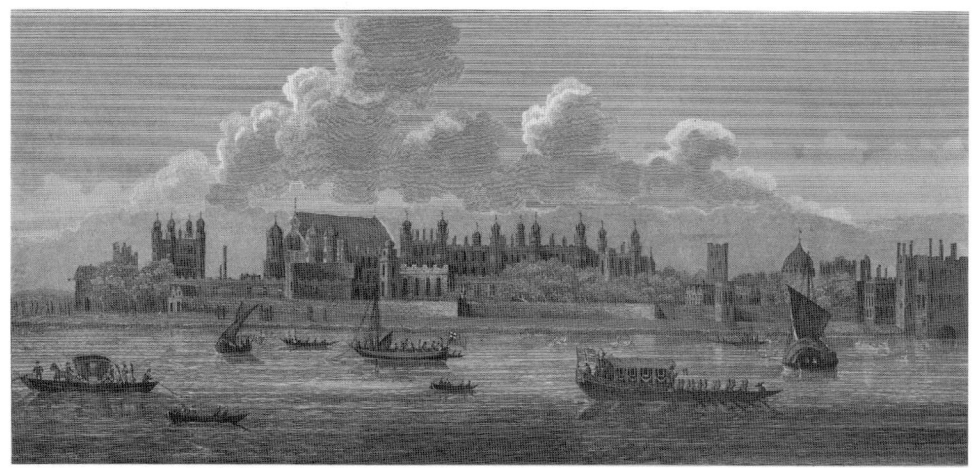

Engraving of the Old Palace at Hampton Court from the Thames by James Basire, 1804. Prince Edward's upbringing was mostly at Hampton Court, where Henry VIII had a self-contained range of buildings erected and special measures put in place to safeguard him from infection. (© *Public Domain: Yale Center for British Art, Paul Mellon Collection*)

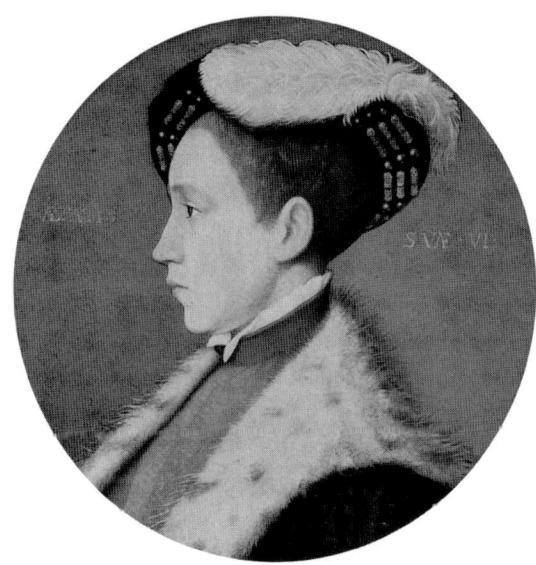

Portrait of Edward as Duke of Cornwall aged six by Hans Holbein the Younger, circa 1545. (© *Stephen Porter*)

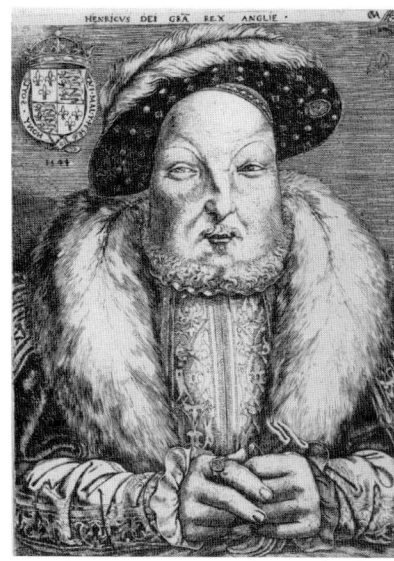

Engraving of Henry VIII by Cornelis Massys, circa 1547. Fear of the sweating sickness was one of the major triggers for Henry's well-known hypochondria. (© *Stephen Porter*)

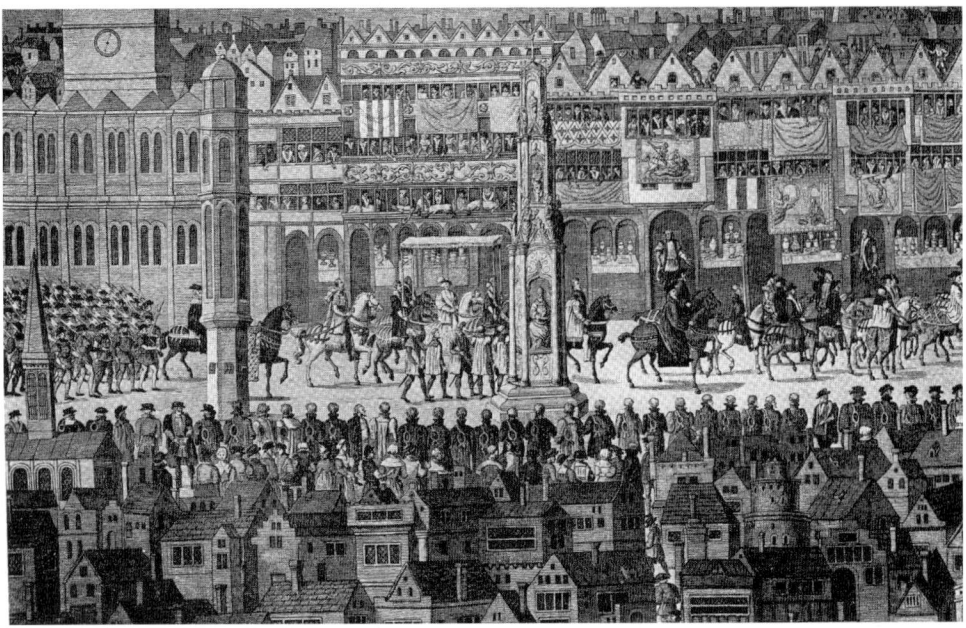

The Coronation procession of Edward VI in 1547 passing through Cheapside in London. (© *Stephen Porter*)

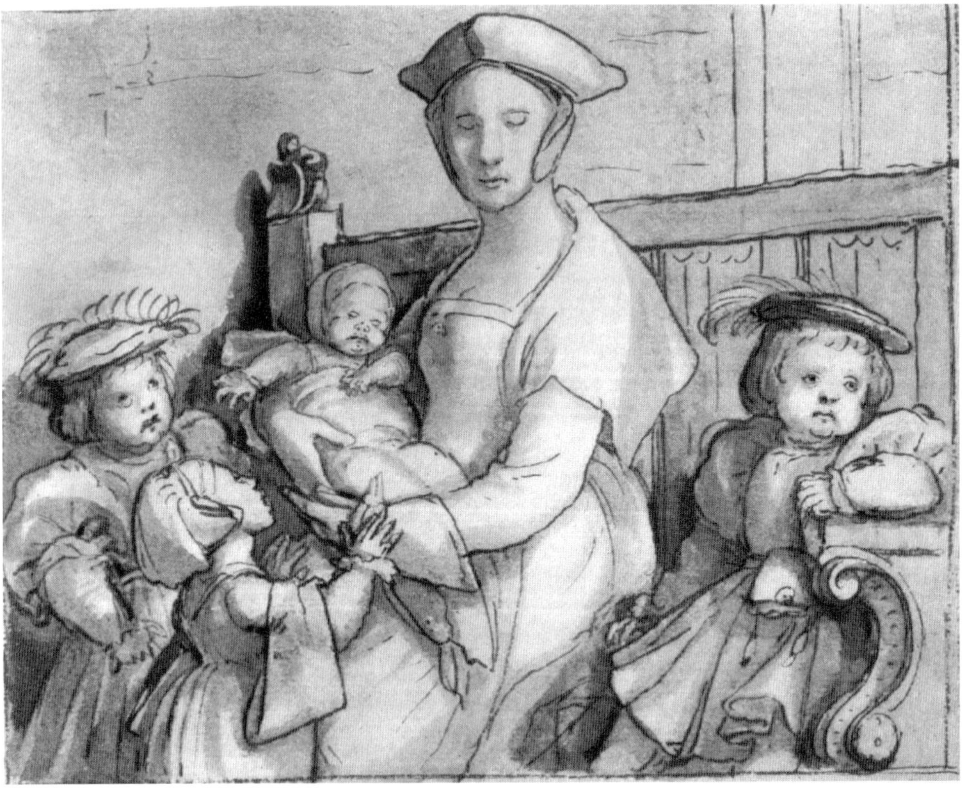

Drawing of the Brandon Family by Hans Holbein the Younger. The teenage Henry and Charles Brandon both died of the sweating sickness in 1549 within half an hour of each other. (© *Stephen Porter*)

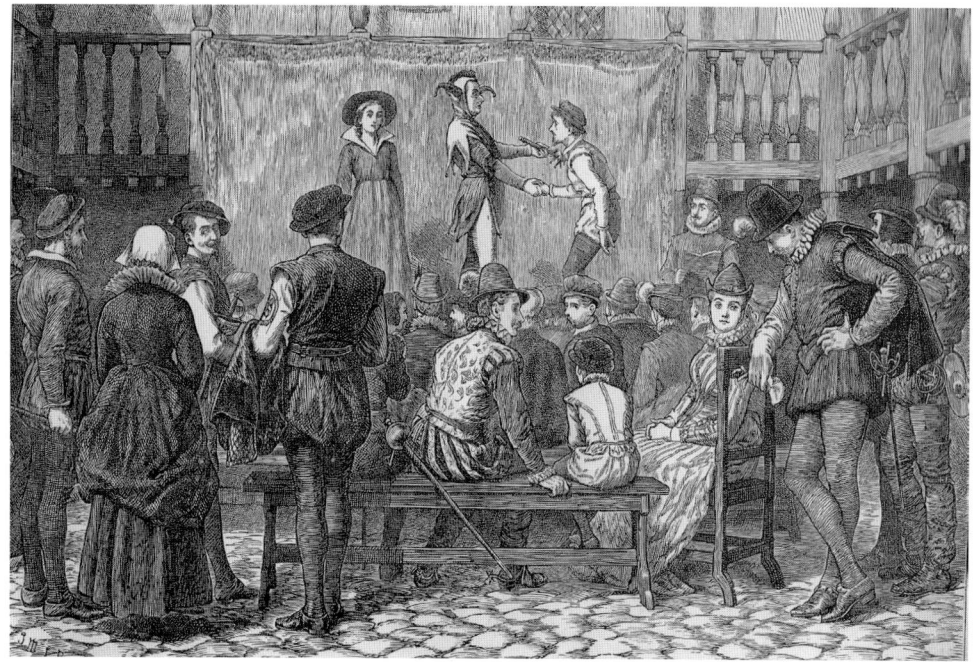

A play performed in the yard of an inn. Audiences crowding together risked the spread of contagion, so plays could be performed only after a licence had been obtained from the Lord Mayor in the City of London. (© *Stephen Porter*)

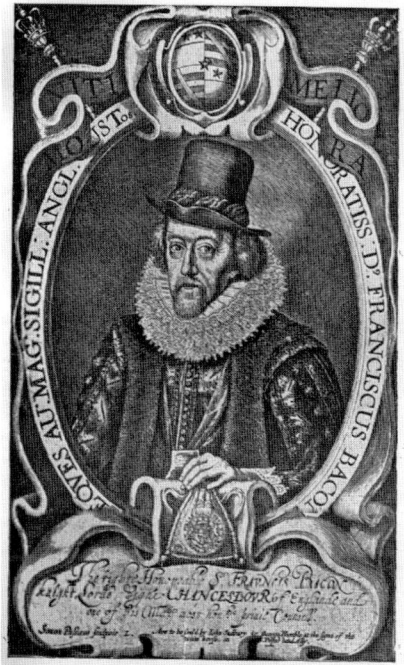

Engraving of Sir Francis Bacon by Simon van de Passe. Bacon wrote a history of the reign of Henry VII. (© *Stephen Porter*)

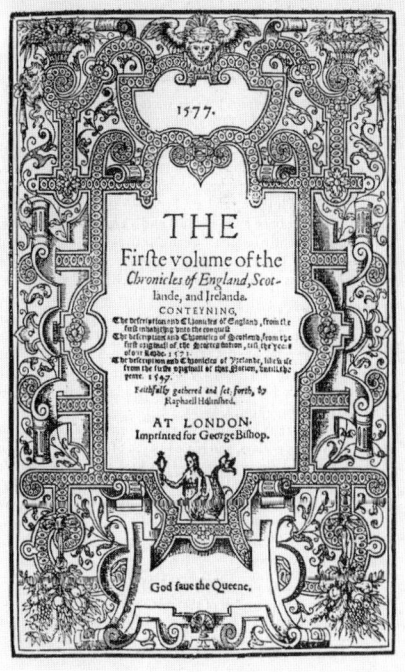

The title page of the Fifth Volume of the Chronicles of England, Scotland and Ireland, 1577, by Raphael Holinshed. (© *Stephen Porter*)

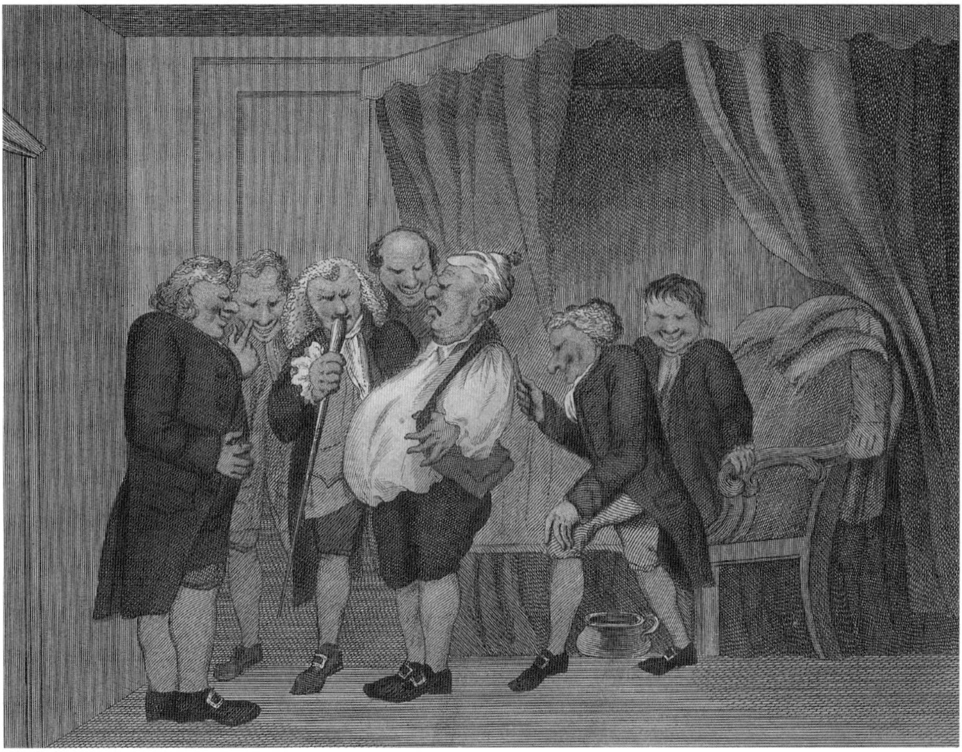

Cartoon showing Tom Ruby being tricked by six friends into thinking he is suffering from the 'sweating sickness', thereby missing his feast, after John Nixon, 1799. (© *Public Domain: Wellcome Collection*)

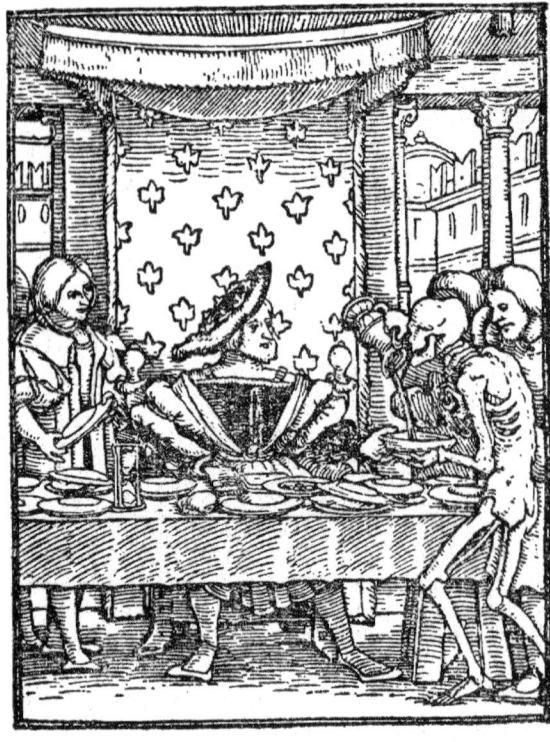

Woodcut from The Dance of Death by Hans Holbein the Younger. The King feasts with his nobles while Death pours his wine. (© *Stephen Porter*)

and went to divers parts of the city inhabited by French and Flemish artificers and mechanics, sacked their houses and wounded many of them, though it was not understood that any were killed'. Giustinian added that they had ransacked the house of the king's French secretary and that they would have killed him if he had not 'escaped up the belfry of the adjoining church'. The houses of Florentine, Lucchese and Genoese merchants were threatened, but were too well defended to be entered. The aldermen's attempts to regain control of the streets were repelled, or ignored, and 'more people arose out of every quarter'. Edward Hall believed that at one point there were 600 or 700 rioters in Cheapside, the City's principal street. The Lieutenant of the Tower was Sir Richard Cholmley, a Yorkshire knight who was hostile to the City. As the fortress was outside its boundary, he did not have jurisdiction there, but evidently felt that some intervention was required to subdue the demonstrators. He ordered that cannon on the Tower's walls should be fired into the City, which was done, although the shot 'did little harm'. The latent threat posed to Londoners by the Tower's artillery had long been recognised, but that was quite different from when it was put into practice, which could only increase the citizens' insecurities. A letter sent to Mantua a few days later mentioned that 'cannon were fired to intimidate the town'. Neither the City authorities nor Cholmley's artillery quelled the disturbance, which was done by the Duke of Norfolk with a force of armed men that dispersed the rioters. In the aftermath 278 people were arrested; 15 of them were executed. Perhaps more humiliating for the aldermen than their failure to maintain law and order in their city was that they had to appear before the king in Westminster Hall dressed in their livery, accompanied by the prisoners with halters around their necks. They pleaded pardon from the king, who graciously granted it to them and 'all that came that time'.[11] Giustinian summarised the riot as 'a great commotion, but the terror was greater than the harm done'. But a nervous Erasmus chose not to return to England in its aftermath and others may have been deterred for a similar reason. The mood in the capital must have been distinctly edgy as the summer approached.

The summer meant celebratory events for the court, which the king was planning when the sweating sickness erupted in July, which according to Hall 'endured ... unto the midst of December'. A letter sent from London on 1 August mentioned that 'a disease is broken out here, causing death within six hours. They call it the sweating sickness. An immense number die of it'. By 6 August Giustinian could report that many of his own household were sick, so that 'the sick outnumber the sound', that few 'strangers' had died but 'an immense number of the natives'. Wolsey had been ill with 'this sweating sickness', from which many of his household had died 'including some of his chief attendants'. The Bishop of Winchester also contracted the disease and the king had left London 'with a few of his attendants to a certain remote and unusual habitation, in consequence of this new malady'. The phrase suggests that Giustinian had not encountered the disease before, and that it had broken out recently.[12]

A letter to the Chief Secretary of the Marquis of Mantua, also written on 6 August, paints a grim picture of conditions in England. According to the writer's summary, in Oxford 'upwards of 400 students had died in less than a week'. The disease was on the increase 'and already circulated throughout the kingdom, the dead being borne to their graves in every direction. Many of the royal household had perished, and several of the household of the cardinal'. Wolsey himself was 'in the country, where, according to report, he, together with his chief attendants, were sweating'. The king and queen, too, 'were gone with a few attendants to healthier places'. Thomas More wrote to Erasmus on 19 August with the news from London, which was not good: 'If ever we were in trouble before, our distress and danger are at their greatest now, with many deaths on all sides and almost everyone in Oxford and Cambridge and London taking to their beds within a few days and the loss of many of my best and most honourable friends'. He and his wife were unscathed, but the disease had afflicted some members of his household, who had recovered. This suggests that the Mores themselves had not ventured out, but those who went to market and the shops to obtain the necessary supplies had done so as usual and had contracted the malady. Other well-to-do householders probably acted in that way, quarantining themselves at home but being cared for by servants who had to go out. More's rather pessimistic opinion that 'one is safer on the battlefield than in the city' surely reflected the mood that the epidemic had produced. Indeed, the atmosphere of dread that the epidemic created was such that 'very few were those who did not fear for their lives, whilst some were so terrified by it that they suffered more from fear than others did from the sweat itself'. By 12 August Giustinian updated his earlier report with the news that both he and his son had caught the disease, that Wolsey had 'suffered the disease three times in a few days; many of his attendants had died, and most especially his gentlemen' and that in London all was silent. Giustinian's colleague Niccolò Sagundino had also caught the sweat and recovered from it before the end of August. On the other hand, by 19 August 'many men of great note' had succumbed to the disease.[13]

Within a few days, Wolsey met Giustinian to discuss diplomatic business, so evidently recovery from the sickness was quite rapid, for those who survived. But by 27 August Giustinian again found himself thwarted because the King was at Windsor, 'alone with his physician, [Dionysius] Memo, and three of his favourite gentlemen; nor does he admit any one, for fear of this disease'. Dionysius Memo was a distinguished organist who had arrived at court from Venice the previous September 'with a most excellent instrument of his' and quickly established himself as the king's favourite musician. He had resigned his place as organist of St Mark's so that he could join Henry's court. The king was both a discerning listener to music and a practising musician himself, and other musicians from the Italian states were persuaded, at different times, to come to England, where they formed a distinct unit at court. In the 1520s five of the seven Italians in the king's shawm and sackbut consort were Venetians. Memo presumably was chosen as one of the king's small and itinerant party to provide musical solace for Henry as he moved from place to place; travelling with the king gave Memo some protection from the sweat, for the monarch was more securely protected than anyone else and that security extended to members of his entourage. Even so, it could not have been a comfortable position for Memo to find himself in and he may have reflected that he had evaded the plague in Venice only to encounter the sweating sickness in England.

The sickness was 'now making very great progress in the land, so that many of those who accompanied the King have died, and it is said that his majesty means to change his quarters'. There had not been such changing of accommodation by a pared-down royal party since the latter stages of Henry VII's reign. The king's choice of residences had been reduced by the fire in the apartments of Westminster palace in 1512. Business became more difficult and protracted when Wolsey, who had been ill with the sickness four times, announced that he was off to Walsingham in Norfolk on a pilgrimage of thanksgiving for having survived the malady; his appearance was said to have shown how much the disease had affected him.[14] The Michaelmas law term was cancelled and at the Inner Temple there were no readings in the autumn vacation 'because of the great plague of the sweating sickness'.[15] Not only did the absence of the king and Wolsey impair the conduct of business, but the very news of conditions in England was a deterrent to diplomats and merchants. Luigi d'Aragona, known as the Cardinal of Aragon, had planned to visit the king and had reached Calais with his impressive retinue, which included 40 horses, but he turned back because of the plague in England, sending on a letter to Wolsey. Sir Richard Wingfield, the Deputy in Calais, told him that 'large numbers in that island [England] were dying of a disease they call the sweating sickness because it kills by making men sweat, within 24 hours at the most, and is highly contagious, and that in London, the capital of that kingdom, 500 had died of it in a day'. In any case, an audience with the king would have been difficult, because he 'keeps aloof at Windsor to avoid the sickness'. He was probably as relieved as was the cardinal, for entertaining such an important figure and his entourage would have been difficult in such circumstances. This was a case of deploying the news of an outbreak of the sweating sickness for diplomatic purposes.[16]

Among the other courtiers, Thomas Lord Clinton, who died on 7 August, and Lord Grey of Wilton were among those who succumbed.

The young Lord Grey was described as 'late the King's henchman' and his burial cost of £10 was paid out of the royal purse. The king's Latin Secretary, Erasmus's friend Andreas Ammonius, was another victim. According to More, Ammonius had not moved away because he believed that his lifestyle gave him protection, even though he admitted that he rarely met anyone 'whose whole household had not suffered'; he was holding to that view until a few hours before he went down with the sweat. When he realised that he was infected he made his will, on 17 August, and died during the night, eight hours after he exhibited the symptoms. He was buried on 19 August.[17] Among the letters of sympathy was one from the Pope, and there was regret that this accomplished man, who was about 40 years old, had not lived to reach the high rank which, contemporaries thought, he surely would have done.

The contemporary accounts suggest that the sweat broke out in London before the end of July, was rampant during most of August, when many died, and receded by September. Giustinian told his masters in Venice on 20 September that he had left London to avoid the plague, and it is most unlikely that he made a slip and meant the sweat, or misidentified the disease. The main substance of his report was a threat of an insurgency in London, which he described as 'another conspiracy formed by the populace for the purpose of cutting all the strangers to pieces and sacking their houses'. He suggested that this had arisen because of the power vacuum created by the absence of the king, Wolsey and other 'lords of the kingdom', but reassured his readers with the information that the authorities were prepared (as they had not been for May Day), with 3,000 citizens armed and waiting to be called out and three suspected ringleaders detained. A letter of 15 October to Wolsey referred to the fear of the 'great plague'. Giustinian mentioned the plague again on 11 November, when he wrote that Wolsey had returned to London for two days 'and as the plague was making great progress, went back to a certain place of his, where he will remain until after Christmas'. The king was still moving from place to place with his few companions and 'all business, both public and private, has on this account been postponed'. It seems that the epidemic of the sweating sickness in the summer was followed that autumn by an outbreak of plague that was serious enough to again alarm the king and disrupt the court and government. On 22 December Giustinian wrote that 'Universal complaints are heard on account of the absence of the court, which is occasioned solely by fear of the plague, which has now abated somewhat'. No doubt his own frustrations at not being able to pursue the matters which he was instructed to discuss with the English government partly prompted his reaction, but there was no doubt that the second half of 1517 had been seriously disrupted by the sweating sickness and then the plague, and that would have applied to commercial business as well as to the government of the realm. That interruption continued into January 1518, with Wolsey promising to return to London after the 22nd of the month 'his presence being required for the despatch of many affairs of state, of which his lordship is sole arbiter', while the court remained dispersed.[18] The king had 'kept no solemn Christmas, willing to have no resort for fear of infection'. Beyond the king and the court, it had been a sickly time, a point made by Hall, who attributed the high mortality to the sweat rather than the plague and wrote that 'in some one town half the people died, and in some other town the third part, the Sweat was so fervent and infectious'.[19]

In the atmosphere of imminent danger, to the monarch and the people, the need to introduce some measures became pressing. The Italian states had instituted regulations virtually from the onset of the Black Death in the late 1340s, which were developed during the late Middle Ages until they became a coherent policy designed to prevent the plague breaking out in a community and to regulate behaviour if it did so. The English court could not have been unaware of such precautions and regulations, especially those restricting trade by enforcing orders for ships to observe a 40-day quarantine. English merchants' operations had been affected, links with the Italian states were strong and senior English figures travelled to Italy and were educated there. Italian merchants in London and the group of Italian scholars centred on the Bishop of Worcester, which overlapped with the humanist circle in north-west Europe, could have provided information on the rules implemented during an epidemic.

The most obvious first step for the government to take when plague threatened was to ban shipping from abroad from landing at English ports. That was done by Edward III during the Black Death, albeit too late to be effective as it was not implemented until the plague was already raging across much of the country. News from abroad that was received and acted upon in good time was crucial if that policy were to work. It would not apply in the case of the sweating sickness, because the outbreaks of the disease began in England and so action was limited to restricting its spread internally by containing it where it was identified. Preventing internal trade was a difficult policy to enforce, as it would conflict with all sorts of economic imperatives, not least the supply of food to urban populations. To overcome that problem the use of health certificates had become common in western Europe, with travellers issued with a document stating that the area from which they had come was free from the disease. In practice, that was open to abuse through forgery, but it did meet the objections of those who were aware of the potential impact of a complete travel ban, and its widespread adoption suggests that the certificates were generally accepted as being authentic.

Household quarantine was also deployed, to restrict infected householders and their contacts to their own houses. Ordering victims and those suspected of being infected with the disease to remain at home required the co-operation of those who were quarantined, who would need provisions for their sustenance and would hardly be willing to starve rather than be disobedient and go out to obtain supplies. That was accepted and the solution adopted was that those who left an infected house carried a white rod so that passers-by could identify them and give them a wide berth. With a range of measures already in place in many European states, not just the Italian ones, which had been honed by usage, it might be thought easy for the English government to have abandoned laissez-faire. Yet changing a previous policy at a time when circumstances were invariably difficult and the citizens fraught with anxiety may have led to opposition on a scale which the government would find hard to deal with. As with other social policies, general cooperation or acquiescence was required if they were to be effective. The sweating sickness had the added difficulty of the speed with which it spread; by the time that the problem had been identified and orders issued, the disease could have been beyond control and already have swept through a town.

Despite the difficulties, on 26 September 1517, the king sent a letter to the Dean and Chapter of St George's College at Windsor pointing out that beggars and other infected persons were entering the college and taking the clothing of those who had been infected. He required them to put an end to the practice. Given the king's visits to Windsor at that time, that may have been prompted by the need to protect his person. Their response was to order that regular searches should be made to ensure that there were no 'strange persons' lodging in the college's houses, who had come from London or any other place where the infection was present. Any resident who became infected was to remain indoors in their house, not receive visitors and only go out to obtain 'meat and drink and other necessaries' and then to carry a white rod at least four feet long, held upwards; they were to do that while there was infection at the house and then for 40 days after the last infection there. The houses that were shut up in this way were to be distinguished by a wisp of straw or hay hung out on a pole at least eight feet long. The order was issued on 1 November and contained the beginning of the practice of household quarantine, which became the basis of the English plague orders as developed during the sixteenth century, albeit they concerned a single closed community under royal supervision.[20]

A few months later a royal proclamation was issued that contained the basis of policy for epidemics. That was done on Wolsey's orders. On 13 January 1518, London householders whose houses were infected with disease (and presumably both plague and the sweating sickness were intended), should put a pole 10 feet long with straw on the end projecting from the building on the side facing the street. It was to be kept on the house for 40 days after the last appearance of the disease, identifying it as one to be avoided. The rule was maintained that anyone who went out of the house was to carry a white rod four feet long. Furthermore, a plague victim's clothes were not to be worn for three months after their death. Those simple measures very much resemble the ones devised for St George's College, which presumably provided the basis for them, although they do not mention beggars. That did not reflect an oversight on the part of the council, for mendicants were the subject of attention during those years and in 1518 a new appointment was made by the City, of an official whose duties included searching for able vagabonds and beggars; the infirm and the elderly were classified as the 'impotent' beggars and were to be licensed to beg. But three weeks after the proclamation in January some citizens 'not only contempted' the proclamation 'but also have murmured and grudged and also have had seditious words whereby commotion or rebellion might arise within this city'.[21] That may have reflected the continuation of the discontent in the city which had erupted on May Day and had threatened again in the autumn, combined with resentment of the imposition of rules for the common householders to obey at a time of extreme social stress. Yet there was a determination in the government, promoted by Wolsey, to persist with the policy and similar orders to those contained in the royal proclamation were issued by Thomas More in Oxford, when the king was at Abingdon. They were summarised as requiring 'that the inhabitants of those houses that be and shall be infected shall keep in, put out wisps and bear white rods, according as your grace [Wolsey] devised for Londoners'. He added that the inhabitants of Oxford were 'right well contented to observe' the order. On 28 April More reported that three children had died of the plague in Oxford 'but none others'. The king referred the matter to the council, which approved More's action and debated the advisability of cancelling the forthcoming fair at Oxford. The argument in favour of cancellation was that if the fair went ahead the traders and others from London who went to it would make Oxford as dangerous as the capital itself. Yet there was the reservation that Londoners would react badly to the fair not being held and would see it as a restriction on their trade. Essentially, if the fair were prevented 'there should ensue grudges and murmurs amongst the King's subjects; especially in London, where they would think that men went about utterly to destroy them, if, with other their misfortunes, they should also be kept from their fairs and markets'. That argument won the day and the council 'after great debating' decided not to prohibit the fair; fears of alienating London's volatile traders had carried more weight than pursuing a measure that would restrict the spread of contagious disease.[22] That incident goes some way to explaining the difficulty of introducing a plague policy and why that had not been attempted sooner. Some offenders were pursued by the aldermen and punished, but it was instructive that even though Wolsey held more power than anyone in early Tudor England had done, apart from the king, even his attempts met with hostility. They were issued at a difficult time, for it is likely that economic conditions had brought into sharper focus the Londoners' latent hostility to the Flemish and French in the city, which erupted on May Day, and that their resentment lingered on into the New Year, while mortality and the conditions that followed had been very high through the summer and well into the autumn.

The London orders of January 1518 may have been drawn up by the same common hand as those for St George's, Windsor. They were not in themselves innovative. The marking of infected houses had been ordered at Lille in 1480 and in Paris in 1510, also by a wisp of straw. In London the order was changed in 1521 when the straw was to be replaced by a headless cross, known as a St Anthony's cross, again fixed on the front of the building. By 1531 Paris had also changed its marker, to the more substantial wooden cross.[23]

The plague, and possibly the sweating sickness, continued into 1518 and so the king maintained his practice of changing houses. A letter sent to Wolsey in July from Wallingford reported that his majesty was about to leave for Bisham, 'for they do die in these parts in every place, not only of the smallpox and measles, but also of the great sickness'. In February Erasmus told one of his circle that he admired the Bishop of Paris for undertaking a mission to England 'on a painful subject, to treat with the English, in winter, and not least when everything over there is raging with a new kind of pestilence'. Presumably, that was a reference to the sweating sickness. He added that 'in England nothing is safe from the plague'. In March he asked a friend to look after a servant of his during a visit to England: 'Please assist him to find a wagon and reliable company ... In default of any other place, take him into your own house, so that he is not obliged to set foot in inns, which are now under suspicion everywhere'.[24] During the summer the king and queen were equally anxious for the other's safety, especially to avoid the danger that London posed. Katherine was insistent that Henry should not go there and is reported to have said that 'though she be no prophet, yet she would lose her finger if some inconvenient should not ensue unto the king's person if he should at this time repass towards London'.[25]

By the summer Giustinian had had enough and on 22 July he wrote to the Signory of Venice asking to be relieved of his post. Over the previous year or so he had found access to Wolsey to be difficult, and he did not like the cardinal, and so doing business had become quite complicated. With the threatening atmosphere in London, Giustinian was glad of an opportunity to get away. He pointed out that he had been in England for 44 months 'and within the last few days two of my servants have died of plague in the house, and I have had the sweating sickness twice in one week'. Plague had rumbled on through the winter months and increased in its virulence again in the summer of 1518, and the sweating sickness had returned, perhaps in a less deadly form than before. On 29 July the Pope's legate Cardinal Lorenzo Campeggio reached London, which he entered 'really in very stately form, save that neither King nor Cardinal [Wolsey] were present, for dread of infection'. This emphasised the disruptive impact of epidemic disease on normal practices, and on the king's dignity, for etiquette and the grandeur of the English state demanded that he, as monarch, should welcome such an important figure as a papal legate to the country. Meanwhile, Giustinian still had work to do: 'Should the Cardinal of York [Wolsey] have dismissed his fear of infection of the plague, I will endeavour to negotiate the matters which remain.'[26] Yet he did not get away until almost the end of July 1519. During his final few months, he did not mention in his despatches the plague or the sweat as disruptive factors and it seems that their threat had receded; they caused far fewer deaths during the remainder of the decade than they had done during the torrid years of 1517 and 1518.

Chapter Six

The Outbreaks of 1528 and 1529

Neither the sweating sickness nor plague aroused undue anxiety in the early 1520s, and so no further regulations were issued. Nor were any additional practices devised to protect the king should there be an epidemic. Dispersal of the courtiers and the isolation of the monarch with as few people as possible remained the procedure to be followed. The size of the court was increased in 1525 when the Princess Mary and her illegitimate half-brother Henry Fitzroy were given administrative responsibilities in Wales and the Marches and Yorkshire respectively, supported by new households. Mary's household numbered 304 in July 1525 and Henry's was roughly the same size.[1] Both would need to be protected and their households provided for or dispersed if an epidemic struck.

While the need for the sovereign to be safe from threatening diseases must have been understood, he was also expected to maintain the normal level of hospitality and be seen by his subjects. Long-term seclusion could meet with disapproval. That could be a fine line and Hall described how at Christmas 1525:

> In this winter was great death in London, wherefore the [legal] term was adjourned, and the king for to eschew the plague, kept his Christmas at Eltham with a small number, for no man might come thither, but such as were appointed by name: this Christmas in the king's house, was called the still Christmas. But the Cardinal in this season lay at the Manor of Richmond, and there kept open household, to lords, ladies, and all other that would come, with plays and disguising in most royal manner: which sore grieved the

people, and in especial the king's servants, to see him keep an open Court, and the king a secret Court.[2]

Christmas was the festive season when the citizens could wander through the palaces and marvel at the rich furnishings and decorations; being prevented from doing so that year clearly rankled. The implication was that the king's popularity fell somewhat as a result and the cardinal's rose because of their contrasting behaviour at the most enjoyable feast of the year. Part of the resentment may have come from a general awareness that the late December of a plague year was a low point for the disease, which peaked in the summer and autumn, before its incidence declined. The commoners would have known that and have expected the king's entourage to have been aware of the pattern, too, and so have relaxed access to the king and royal houses at that time of the year rather than keep it so tightly controlled. Wolsey was not a popular chief minister and was seen as avaricious of power, positions, status and wealth, and far too proud for a clergyman. He had effectively supplanted the queen in political influence and her failure to produce a male heir further reduced her sway with the king.

Cause for concern continued into 1526, when the king's route to Winchester in July was changed because one of the houses in which he was to have lodged was infected with plague. To those who could remember the previous decade, this would have been familiar, but the political situation had changed dramatically since then, and the king's progresses reflected that. Fearful that the queen was unable to bear a son, and that their marriage was unlawful, at least in the eyes of God, because she had earlier been married to his brother, the king began to look around for a solution to the Tudor dynastic problem. He became drawn to Anne Boleyn, a lady of the court who had spent time in Mechelen and Paris and knew the ways of the court. She was determined to play for the highest stakes and would not yield to the king's desires until he promised to make her queen. That, of course, would mean divorcing, or rather annulling, his marriage to Katherine, who was adamant that she would not comply and go quietly. Henry appealed to the Pope, Clement VII, but he could see no reason why the divorce was necessary and in any case, he was not a free agent, for in 1527 the troops of Katherine's nephew, the Emperor Charles V, occupied and sacked Rome. Charles would not consent to his aunt being treated other than as she wished. Henry was so far committed to his course of action that he made it clear that unless he had his own way he would separate the English church from its allegiance to Rome. The stakes could hardly have been higher and the Pope sought to find a way out of the impasse by appointing Cardinal Wolsey, Henry's Chancellor, and Cardinal Campeggio, absentee Bishop of Salisbury, as his legates to find a solution. With the papacy under Imperial control, Campeggio was subject to political pressure not to agree to the divorce and to delay the proceedings. He had to make his way from Rome to London, stricken by painful attacks of gout. When he arrived, the king, Campeggio and his officials would have to be accommodated safely and near to each other. It was decided that Henry and his entourage were to be lodged at Bridewell Palace and the hearings would be held in the hall of the Blackfriars monastery. A wooden gallery had been built to connect the two buildings for the visit of Charles V in 1522, when Henry VIII and his party lodged at Bridewell; that insulated those who had to pass between the buildings from the potentially unsanitary and infectious crowds in the London streets.

There was some disquiet at the English court in the early summer of 1528 when Campeggio had failed to even reach France; it was a bad season for plague in southern Europe, and then, to add to the accumulating anxiety, the sweating sickness broke out in England 'beginning in the end of May, and continuing [through] June and July'.[3] Edward Hall put the start of the epidemic at 'the very end of May'; the legal term was postponed on 17 June, to begin again at Michaelmas, 29 September, and the assizes were cancelled. Reports sent to Venice informed the Signory in late July that no business could be transacted with the English court because neither the king nor Wolsey were available, but towards the end of August the disease was said to have been much reduced. That suggests that the epidemic lasted for roughly three months and Hall wrote that England 'all this summer season had been troubled and vexed with the sweating sickness' which had begun in London 'and afterward went all the realm almost'. John Stow noted that 'Many died in England of the sweating sickness, in especially about London'.[4]

The court had been taken by surprise and the Boleyn household had not taken evasive action soon enough to escape the disease. One of Anne's ladies contracted it and the family retreated to the relative seclusion of Hever Castle in Kent, 30 miles from London. Anne believed that 'those who keep a good diet' were less likely to suffer, but both she and her father, Sir Thomas, caught the disease. The king wrote to reassure her, with the comments that 'few women have this illness; and moreover none of our court and few elsewhere have died of it'. Neither statement was correct and in the same letter, he admitted that some members of the royal household had contracted the malady, but had recovered, and in a later missive he confessed that five men, including an apothecary, 'are fallen of the sweat in this house' and all had recovered. The king was not the best source of advice. He told Sir Brian Tuke, Wolsey's chief secretary and Clerk of the Parliament, 'how little danger there was if good order be observed; how few were dead of it' and recommended that everyone should eat 'small suppers' and drink little wine. Both Anne and her father survived the attack (contemporaries must subsequently have wondered how things might have developed had she died at that time), but her brother-in-law William Carey, her sister Mary's husband, and his fellow courtier Sir William Compton did not escape and both died in June.[5] So did Sir Francis Poyntz, erstwhile ambassador to Spain, who died in London; a letter to Wolsey of 26 June noted only that 'Poynes is dead'. It reflected the nature of the times that the death of a man of such standing should be mentioned so tersely.[6]

The alarm among the elite was widespread. On 5 June Sir Brian Tuke wrote that he had fled to Stepney 'for fear of this infection, a servant of mine being ill at my house in London'. The Bishop of Lincoln told Wolsey that he had remained in his London house while many were dying of the sweat and 'tarried till it came to my house, and then was forced to flee'. The Bishop of Exeter wrote to the cardinal with his best wishes that 'God preserve you from the pestilent air about London'. The Milanese ambassador had left his lodgings 'in great haste because two or three had been suddenly attacked'. The French cardinal and diplomat Jean du Bellay reported that the king 'shuts himself up quite alone. It is the same with Wolsey. But when all is said, those who do not expose themselves to the air rarely die'. According to du Bellay, the king 'keeps moving about for fear of the plague. Many of his people have died of it in three or four hours'. And he added the names of three men who had died and eleven more 'and those of the Chamber generally' who had the disease 'some of them were said to be dead'. He went on to explain that the king had eventually chosen to lodge at one of Wolsey's houses 20 miles from London 'finding removals useless', where he had made his will and taken the sacraments 'for fear of sudden death', while the cardinal had 'stolen away with a very few people, letting no one know where he has gone'. A letter from Hunsdon, in Hertfordshire, dated 23 June, reported that 'the King's grace is very merry since he came to this house, for there was none fell sick of the sweat since he came hither'. Yet he no longer had Dionysius Memo to sweeten his travels. Memo had left England, probably in 1525, and travelled to Santiago de Compostela, in Spain, leaving under a cloud for having been suspected of passing information to the Venetians. The king was uncertain at one stage how Wolsey was faring 'as there are many flying tales that your people are sick', but he did not wish for a meeting because of the risk of infection. Bishop Cuthbert Tunstall needed to see Wolsey but did not dare do so 'as nearly all his servants are troubled with the sweat' and at one point 13 of them had been sick at the same time. When the king was settled at Tyttenhanger in early July he sent a message to the cardinal telling him that 'himself, the Queen, and all others here are well, and the plague so far ceased that none have had the sweat these three days, except Mr. Butt. He is very desirous for your health, and that you will put aside all fear and phantasies, make as merry as you can, put apart all cares for the time, and commit all to God'. The routine for the king's safety at Tyttenhanger was that 'the place was so purged daily with fires and other preservatives, that neither he nor the queen nor none of their company was infected with that disease'. Yet the king was not happy with his security there and soon afterwards moved to Ampthill.[7]

Richard Broke, at Sutton in Kent, excused himself from a visit to Wolsey because he had the sweat. One of his clerks in London had recovered from the disease and another who had written letters for him on the previous day had subsequently fallen ill with it, which showed how quickly and unexpectedly it struck. On 1 July du Bellay wrote that the disease had begun to diminish but was still prevalent in Kent, where 'Divers have been sick at Greenwich and at Eltham; of which towns great numbers would have appeared if the sessions had been held, with other prisoners from Southwark'. His own experience had been horrific: he had contracted the disease while at the Archbishop of Canterbury's palace and while he sweated 18 people died there in the space of four hours, 'and hardly anybody escaped but myself, who am not yet quite strong again'.[8] His news of the decline of the disease was premature but by early August the king was confident enough to plan to be back at Windsor on the 11th, making the return to business easier. There was still Cardinal Campeggio's visit to arrange. By 21 August it was assumed that he was past Lyons and well on his way to Paris. Sir Francis Brian was sent to France to meet him, preferably before he reached Calais, and he was to be asked 'to send a gentleman of his privy chamber hither into England to see, know and understand of the prosperous estate and health of them both; which (lauds be given unto God!) have escaped the great and furious danger of the pestilent plague of sweat lately visiting the realm of England; which plague at this day is well assuaged, and little or nothing heard thereof in any place'.[9]

That may have been rather optimistic, but the disease had subsided by the end of August, and people began to take stock. The king can only have been dismayed at the deaths of two of his long-term friends, Sir William Compton and William Carey, and alarmed by Anne Boleyn's illness. Compton was the son of a Warwickshire landowner who had risen to prominence solely through the king's favour and friendship. Early in the reign, he was appointed to the key position of Groom of the Stool, which put him in daily contact with the king and allowed him to control access to him. Through Henry's favour he accumulated profitable and influential posts and at one time was spoken of as a potential rival to Wolsey for the king's support: he amassed a large estate in the Midlands. He was removed from his position as Groom of the Stool in Wolsey's reform of the royal chamber in 1526, known as the Eltham Ordinances, but had not lost the king's approval. William Carey was among the king's companions and a member of the household by 1519, gambling and playing tennis with him. His marriage to Mary Boleyn, Anne's sister, in 1520 strengthened his social position and his standing at court; he steadily acquired land, was granted a number of positions and survived the purges of the chamber in the Eltham Ordinances, being appointed as one of just six Gentleman Waiters of the privy chamber. He died on 22 June 1528 and Compton eight days later, both succumbing to the sweating sickness.[10]

The Duke of Richmond had taken refuge at Sheriff Hutton in Yorkshire, where he had spent the summer 'without any peril of the rageous sweat that hath reigned in these parts'. The members of the London Carthusian priory, on the other hand, apparently had not dispersed in time and the house had lost four priests and two lay brethren. The disease also claimed prominent victims on the other side of the increasingly acrimonious religious divide, including Francis Denham, who was described as 'a personage of goodly fashion, and marvellously well learned, both in Latin and Greek, but was also right excellent in musical instruments', and Henry Summers, who died at Cardinal College, Oxford (later Christ Church). A report from Oxford at the beginning of September declared that 'The university is little infected but there [that college]. Our Lord preserve it!' By then four victims of the sweat who were regarded as heretics had died and had attracted the wrath of the dean even after their deaths, for they 'were buried in Christian sepulture, but the sacrament was denied them by the dean'.[11]

Du Bellay thought that there had been an urgent hurry to make wills, in anticipation of imminent death, and that the notaries had done well financially as a result: 'I think 100,000 wills have been made off-hand, for those who were dying became quite foolish the moment they fell ill'.

Those who were afraid that they had contracted the sweat could be seen 'as thick as flies hurrying out of the streets and the shops into the houses, to take the sweat the instant they were seized by the distemper'. That is, they were rushing home to wrap themselves up and get hot, to try to sweat out the disease. Du Bellay added that 'the priests there have a better time of it than the physicians', presumably referring to fees received for burials, and not for treatments, because the disease acted so quickly. He explained that there had not been an outbreak like it for 12 years and then 10,000 had died within 10 or 12 days. Those who had observed victims, or claimed special knowledge, distributed prescriptions with which victims of the disease could be dosed. The Countess of Norfolk had been banished by the king for too strongly taking the queen's side in the dispute over the annulment and she had gone to Kenninghall, the Norfolks' mansion in the county, from where she offered advice and remedies. The king himself drew up prescriptions and recommendations. But the concoctions required ingredients that were not available to most people because of their cost and they would have required an apothecary to prepare them. Du Bellay's description of people rushing home to put themselves in a sweat reflected the experience of most people, rather than the ingesting of specialist medicines and pills. In Tuke's opinion fear caused by news of the disease had afflicted many people, who were not otherwise ill, so that some children were put at risk because their mothers kept them too hot if they saw that they were sweating. Fear of the malady produced actions which generated its symptoms and, in his opinion, many fell ill through fear of the disease, so that when a man in good health came from London and talked of the sweat 'the same night all the town is full of it, and thus it spreads as the fame runs'. But he did not deny that there was an infection that was 'greatly to be feared and avoided, which cannot be, if men meet together in great companies in infect airs and places'. Tuke faced reality rather than a phantom disease when his wife contracted the malady. She survived, which Tuke described as having 'passed the sweat', but she was left very weak.[12]

The epidemic had affected much of the country and made inroads into the royal household, had caused the king and his chief minister almost to lose contact with each other, seen sundry bishops on the roads in search of safe havens, and councillors meeting in a field on horseback shouting to each other. Such an outbreak might have prompted further regulations in its aftermath. It did not. Yet it did prompt estimates of numbers. Du Bellay wrote that of the 40,000 infected in London, only 2,000 had died. And returns were made of the number of dead in the city. That for 6-14 August has survived and shows that in that period 'which be 8 days complete, there be dead within the city of London, of the plague and otherwise the full number of 152 persons'. A subsequent return was promised. That figure would have produced a total of deaths in London during the epidemic of just below 2,000. Whether the collection of the figures was initiated by the government or by the City, it was an important development, for if such returns were produced consistently, then an increase in the number of deaths recorded should indicate the imminent onset of an epidemic. That was potentially an important tool for combatting the effects of plague epidemics.[13] Even so, the speed with which the sweating sickness appeared would have been too fast for such an analysis to be made. An indication of the suddenness of the disease's onset was given by du Bellay, who recalled that he was talking with Wolsey in the gardens at Hampton Court when, in the middle of their conversation, news was brought to Wolsey that five or six of his household had 'taken the sweat'. Understandably, their interview was immediately broken off.[14]

Campeggio arrived at Dover on 29 September and in London eight days later, weary and in pain from the gout. He and Wolsey endeavoured to persuade the queen to comply with the king's wishes, but she remained obdurate. Campeggio moved slowly, following his instructions, and when he had recovered from the gout sufficiently to conduct business, towards the end of October the king sent for him and the representatives of France and Venice to discuss what was to be done. That was preceded by mutual congratulations all round at having 'escaped the plague'.[15] But it was not until the following summer that a hearing of the case was opened at Blackfriars. The king and queen both appeared and stated their case, Katherine strongly denying that her marriage to Arthur had been consummated. To the king's frustration, on 31 July Campeggio announced that he was adjourning the hearing until 1 October, because the court was part of the Roman consistory and so would keep the legal terms observed there. It never met again. Wolsey fell from power in October in the aftermath of that debacle. Henry then attempted to obtain his annulment by direct appeals to the Pope and, when they failed, he broke with Rome and assumed the headship of the English church. By chance, and through Campeggio's steady rate of travelling, the case had not been disrupted by the outbreak of sweating sickness in London.

Although no new precautions were put in place in the aftermath of the outbreak, in an important development the collection of information on deaths was extended in the early 1530s and became an established feature of epidemics. In October 1532 the Council ordered the Mayor 'to certify how many have died of the plague' and a return was provided which showed that three-quarters of the 126 recorded deaths across the city were attributed to plague.[16] By then Wolsey's protégé Thomas Cromwell was in the ascendant and had effectively succeeded his former master as the king's chief minister. He asked the Mayor for lists of the victims and the Mayor was indeed able to supply the numbers of those who had died from plague and from other causes. By recording the parishes where plague deaths had occurred, the districts within the capital that were affected could be identified. What was to become the weekly Bills of Mortality were beginning to emerge as a useful tool for the government and the City, with the parish churchwardens given instructions to 'write or cause to be written weekly certificate of all such people as shall die within the City of London and the liberties'.[17] The recording of vital information was extended in 1538 when Cromwell, as Vicar General, ordered that a record be kept of the reading of the services for baptisms, marriages and burials in every parish. Some clerks chose to note the cause of death, especially plague, in their parish register.

In a letter of July 1528, Sir Brian Tuke pointed out that this was an English disease, which in France and Flanders was called the king of England's sickness, 'and is not thought much of there'. He claimed that when the disease was at Calais, which was treated as an English town, it did not spread to Gravelines, along the coast, despite the frequent movements between the two places.[18] That may have been correct when he wrote, but in the following year, an alarming outbreak of the disease in Hamburg was to spread across much of Germany, Austria and the Baltic lands.

The disease was reported to have broken out at Hamburg on 25 July 1529 when a German ship arrived with 12 men on board who were dead or dying. The ship had come from England, the most likely source of infection, which implies a long incubation period, but one which included the dormant winter time. Merchants and sailors who travelled between the two places would have known, indeed been acutely aware of, the symptoms of current diseases and so the identification of the malady as the English Sweat probably was correct. But given that the Hamburg region may have been the source of the epidemic in England in 1485, it does raise the possibility that the English and Hamburg sweating sicknesses had common origins. An epidemic erupted in Hamburg almost immediately after the arrival of the stricken vessel in 1529, with 40 to 60 deaths every day and an extra 1,100 coffins needed within 22 days; estimates put the number of deaths in the outbreak at 1,000 to 1,100. Entries in the records of the cathedral chapter of Lübeck distinguish between 'a great plague' [eine grosse pestilenz] at Hamburg in 1526 and the 'pestis suderosa' [sweating disease] three years later. A chronicle of the history of Eckernförde, in Holstein, noted that in 1529 a 'malignant sweating sickness, also called *sudor anglicus*, killed many people'.[19] A chronicler in Thuringia wrote that 'there was an epidemic of the sweating plague, or English plague, thus named because it came to Germany from England; many thousands of people died suddenly of it; it was such a rapid poison that, if anyone only heard it mentioned and worked himself up into a fright, he died of it', echoing Sir Brian Tuke's opinion that fear led to a phantom malady which contributed to the spread of the disease.[20]

According to John Foxe, the martyrologist, the outbreak coincided with a visit to Hamburg by the theologian William Tyndale, the translator of the Bible into English. He had been living in exile in the Low Countries, rightly fearful for his own safety if he returned to England. According to Foxe, he had hoped to print part of his Old Testament translation in the city but had been shipwrecked between Antwerp and Hamburg and had lost all his materials and his money in the wreck. Nevertheless, he pressed on to Hamburg in another ship, where he met his fellow translator Miles Coverdale, who was waiting there for him. Together they translated the Book of Moses between March and December 1529, lodging in a widow's house, 'a great sweating sickness being the same time in the town'. They escaped the disease and when their task was completed Tyndale returned to Antwerp.[21]

Hamburg was a busy port with a population of around 20,000, trading across the North Sea and into the Baltic and along the rivers within its hinterland of the River Elbe and its tributaries. In 1510 it was declared a Free Imperial City by the Emperor Maximilian, and in 1529 it loosened its restrictions on immigrants, a policy which it maintained thereafter, although more to encourage trade than to provide a safe haven for religious refugees.[22] Trade, rather than religious connections, was no doubt the reason for the rapid spread of the disease through the Baltic. It reached Lübeck on 31 July; no estimates of the numbers were made, but the death toll was reported to be 'unbelievably many in a short time'. It was also said that no children died of the sweat and that the victims were mostly men and women between 16 and 60 years old. Some indication of the increased scale of mortality caused by the virus comes from the number of wills compiled, with three times the number recorded in August than in July. One victim survived to report to the Duke of Mecklenburg how he had been saved. When he realised that he had caught the disease he took some pills of unicorn and gold and went to bed, as was generally recommended, closed the windows, pulled the curtains and lit a roaring fire, so that he felt that he was being roasted to a cinder. But an English merchant had been called in by his friends and he pulled off the bedclothes and quenched the fire. Perhaps he was drawing on practical experience of the sickness in England in the previous year, which was Gilsheim's good fortune, for he survived, and had the accepted practices of sweating out the disease been continued they might have killed him. Hubertus Thomas also survived the ministrations of 'an ignorant knavish doctor' who was the chief medical man in Heidelberg. That physician, according to the common practice, ordered him to keep to his bed for twenty-four hours, without a drop to drink. He was saved by an elderly woman who was aware that he was not being cared for and so gave him a flagon of beer and the advice to take a long draught. Hubertus was so thirsty that he drained it off and almost at once 'sprang out of bed as though there was nothing the matter'.[23]

Bremen was stricken around the same date as Lübeck, Stettin on 31 August and at roughly the same time the sickness erupted in Wismar, Rostock and Stralsund; by 1 September it was at Gdansk, where between 3,000 and 6,000 victims died, and in Königsberg a week later. Copenhagen also experienced an epidemic in 1529, with 400 deaths, as did Elsinore (Helsingör). Scandinavia was also blighted and the virus claimed a royal life there, with the death of Magnus Eriksson, brother of the Swedish king Gustav Wasa. From the ports it spread inland, causing an estimated 30,000 deaths in Prussia, and then across Livonia and Lithuania in 1530 and on into Poland and Russia.[24]

From Hamburg the sweating sickness ran northwards into Schleswig and Holstein and the Danish islands, and inland in Germany to Hanover and Göttingen by the middle of August, infecting Brunswick, Lüneburg, Waldeck, Hadeln, Einbeck, Westphalia, the valley of the Weser and East Friesland. A parallel with the practice of managing large houses in England during an outbreak occurred at the Duke of Mecklenburg's great house at Boizenburg on the Elbe, where the steward reported that he and the bailiff had closed the house and dismissed the staff, retaining only the porter, the cook and a maid. He included the chilling note that in Boizenburg 60 people had died between 10 and 13 August.[25] By 11 September the virus was at Frankfurt and then at Worms; it reached Marburg at the end of the month.

By the late 1520s, the religious reformers had attracted such support that cities and towns were adopting Lutheranism and denying the authority of the Roman Catholic church; Hamburg took that step in 1529. Aware of their vulnerability to a reaction from the establishment, both ecclesiastical and lay, the reformers sought to form closer bonds and reach agreement on doctrinal matters. Philip of Hesse offered his castle at Marburg as a meeting place where the leading reformers, including Martin Luther and Ulrich Zwingli, could debate their differences. The conference went ahead on 1 October and 14 of the 15 points were resolved. Before it broke up on 4 October the doctrines on which there was agreement were summarised and issued as the Marburg Articles. It may have been that even had the delegates stayed longer they would not have reached an accord on the fifteenth point, concerning the nature of the Eucharist, because of their intransigence on that issue. But according to Luther they left prematurely because of the imminent threat of the sweating sickness and had that not reached the district when it did, perhaps the delegates would have stayed on and their discussions might have produced an agreement. The conference was not re-convened and the nature of the Eucharist remained a doctrine that divided the Protestant cause.[26] (Marburg was to give its name to a haemorrhagic fever virus that reached Germany from Uganda in 1967.)

By roughly the middle of September Jülich, Liege and Cologne had been affected and there was a severe epidemic in Augsburg after 6 September, while Strasburg was infected in the last week of that month. At Göttingen it was said that eight corpses had to be buried in one grave so that the speed of interments could be kept up with the number of bodies being delivered for burial. The outbreak at Augsburg was reported to have claimed 800 victims, but despite the speed with which the virus spread the city's printers were able to prepare and print pamphlets that dealt with the crisis. They fell into two broad groups; those that discussed the medical issues and those that addressed the theological implications of the disease. The members of the printing trade who produced the pamphlets clearly thought that the commercial opportunities created by the virus outweighed the advice to move swiftly away to safety. And they judged that enough of the citizens had remained to provide customers for their publications. They were not unique, for at least 21 essays or pamphlets of advice on the disease were printed in Germany, the Netherlands and Switzerland between October 1529 and June 1531. That contrasted with England, where the epidemic produced no such printed response.[27] Their recommendations were, in any case, more encouraging than efficacious; one issued in Antwerp advised trusting in God, lying flat, keeping cool and drinking light tonics.[28]

It was then rather late in the year for the virus; an unusually wet summer had followed a hot and dry May, with a damp, wet and cold spell from midsummer until the last week in August, when the rain eased off, but foggy and unseasonably warm weather followed 'so that it was impossible not to sweat, even if you had gone naked; and with this weather came the disease'.[29] Perhaps the conditions did favour the spread of the virus, which continued to infect places further south through the autumn, including Freiburg in Breisgau, Mühlhausen and Gebweiler in Alsace, in October, and in November Wurtemberg, Baden, the Upper Rhine and the Palatinate. It reached the shores of Lake Constance and in the Swiss cantons was reported at Berne in December (but it produced the low fatality rate of three deaths among 300 infected), and at Basel in January 1530. On 22 September it was at Vienna, where it continued to cause deaths until 14 October, during the Ottoman army's unsuccessful siege of the city. The siege lasted for only three weeks and the Ottomans' failure was due to the appalling state of the roads and countryside caused by the heavy rains, which literally bogged down their siege artillery, and the defenders' capable deployment of their own weaponry, as much as the epidemic. The virus also brought disease and death to Franconia, Thuringia, Saxony, Meissen, Mannsfeld, Halberstadt, Magdeburg, Wittenberg, Brandenburg and Silesia.

As in England, deaths from the disease were seen to be a punishment for heretics. One anecdote from the epidemic in 1529 told of the death of the lord of Friedberg's son from the English Sweat when he returned home from Wittenberg. The priest took the opportunity to tell his congregation in a sermon that this was how God punished the Lutherans and he required them to go to the church the next day and then take part in a procession against the disease. They did so and indeed formed a procession, but it followed the coffin of the dead priest to his grave, for he had died in the night of the English Sweat. Both Catholics and Lutherans took the opportunity to claim that the disease was a punishment sent by God and provoked by their religious opponents. One anonymous tract was even-handed in that respect, stating that the disease – 'which attacks rapidly and speedily kills' – was God's punishment caused by both the Catholics, who had 'so tyrannically persecuted His divine word', and the evangelicals, who had 'accepted it but have disobeyed it'.[30]

The Netherlands also suffered from that outbreak of the disease, although it was not infected directly from England, with which it carried on a considerable trade, but from the Rhineland to the south. The virus reached Deventer on 7 September, Amsterdam on 27 September and Zierikzee, in Zeeland, on 3 October, where the death toll was said to have been very high. At Antwerp 300-400 deaths followed the virus's appearance in the city on 26-27 September; commemorative processions were held there during the 1530s and as late as 1546. Antwerp was then a burgeoning city and port with a population of approximately 55,000 and many trading contacts.[31]

The virus had travelled a long way in the space of a few months. Fridolin Ryff, a chronicler in Basel, wrote that 'a terrible disease spread in the lowlands at Cologne, Mainz, Frankfurt, Speyer, reaching as far as Strasbourg, so that in these places a great many people died, and they called this disease the English Sweat, because it came from England'. His description of the impact of the sickness was similar to accounts of its effect in England, writing that 'whoever was affected by this disease went from life to death in twenty-four hours, for when one was afflicted with the disease, it came with a great poisonous sweating and one sweated to death forthwith, so that countless people died of the disease everywhere ... Some people sat down to table in good health and were carried away dead'.[32]

The sweating sickness did not cross the Alps, perhaps because of the winter weather and the sheer lack of travellers and movement over the mountains to transmit the disease. Nor did it reach France, Spain and Portugal, the Mediterranean basin or the Balkans. As with the outbreak in England in the previous year, it may have rumbled on into the new year, but intermittently and sporadically, without attracting attention. The epidemic which infected much of northern and parts of central Europe in 1529 was the only major outbreak of the sweating sickness on the Continent.

Chapter Seven

The Final Epidemic

The sweating sickness did not appear in England after the outbreak in 1528 until a recurrence in 1533. That was followed by an unprecedentedly long quiescent interval before another epidemic struck, in 1551. One of the social changes during the period was an ending of pilgrimages and the journeys which they entailed, which removed one group of travellers from the highways and inns. They had fallen in number as Protestant ideas became more widely accepted during the 1530s and were brought to an abrupt end by the abolition of the monasteries, in whose care the shrines generally were. The shrine at Walsingham was served by the Augustinian canons of Walsingham Priory, for example. The shrines were closed and their venerated contents were destroyed, while the buildings themselves were allowed to decay, unless sold and re-purposed by lay owners. Pilgrimages to continental shrines also fell away and even without the change in religious observance in England would have become more difficult undertakings in terms of international politics. Erasmus had earlier poured scorn on long-distance pilgrimages, commenting that a man 'leaves wife and children at home, and goes off to Jerusalem or Rome or St James's shrine, where he has no call to be'.[1] He may have been expressing the intellectuals' view, or he may have reflected a growing and more widely held attitude of scepticism to the shrines, their supposed holy contents and their veneration by the public.

Reactions to the sweat remained basically the same whenever an outbreak was identified, or just suspected. Andrew Boorde was writing for an English readership in the early 1540s when he asserted that 'When the plagues of the pestilence or the sweating sickness is in a town or country

... the people flee from the contagious and infectious air; preservations with other counsel of physic notwithstanding'.[2] Nothing devised by the medical profession had been convincing enough to outweigh the fears of those who could depart when the disease threatened, and so they would leave. Plague occurred with some regularity, indeed almost annually, and produced the same response. But during the 1530s the evolution of the political situation and the king's marital arrangements brought a change to the way in which the members of the royal family were protected. Special circumstances required special measures.

The king persisted with his intention to annul his marriage to Katherine and marry Anne Boleyn, who was pregnant by the time that she and Henry married in January 1533. The child was a girl, the future Elizabeth I, and Anne's next pregnancy ended prematurely with a miscarriage. Disappointed with her as a queen and wife, and with the problem of the succession remaining, Henry had their marriage declared invalid and in May 1536 Anne was executed. Annulment of his marriage to Katherine rendered their daughter Mary illegitimate, removing her claim to the throne; at the same time it raised once more the possibility that Henry Fitzroy could be made legitimate, and so in due course succeed his father.

Attention was paid to Henry Fitzroy's safety and his minders were ordered to move him away from danger when plague threatened. Between 1525 and 1529 the boy lived at Sheriff Hutton in Yorkshire as head of the Council of the North. But on one occasion when reports reached Westminster that plague was present near Pontefract, almost 40 miles away, instructions were sent that he should be taken further north, away from the danger. On a later occasion, a similar report of a hazardous plague outbreak saw him recalled to Windsor, where he could be looked after more closely.[3]

Alarmingly, as the expected date of the birth of Anne Boleyn's child approached, in August 1533 sweating sickness again appeared, sending the king scampering around the palaces and houses to the west of London. He had been in the best of moods recently, hunting deer as a cheerful pastime, which prompted Sir John Russell to write to Lord

Lisle on 6 August that he had never known the king to be merrier. But because of the sweat, he had changed his itinerary, which had been 'to go to Farnham, from thence to East Hampstead, and so to Windsor', but he was now to leave Guildford to go to Sutton and 'within these eight days he cometh again to Windsor, and soon after the Queen removes thence to Greenwich to take her chamber [to prepare for the birth]'. Henry explained to Charles V's ambassador Eustace Chapuys that because one of his physicians and other members of his chamber had been afflicted by the sweat he could not grant him an interview, but Chapuys could meet members of his council who would then report to him. Chapuys pursued this idea and discovered that the king was at 'a private house with none but those of his chamber'. He spoke with Thomas Cromwell (now effectively the king's chief minister), the Bishop of Winchester and the Dean of the Chapel Royal, who passed on his message to Henry. The caution was understandable, for two officers of the king's household had died, and five days later the minister of Waverly, in south-west Surrey, admitted that 'we are troubled in these parts with the sweat'. On the other side of London Sir Thomas Audley, Speaker of the House of Commons and Keeper of the Great Seal, wrote from Colchester on the last day of August to report that he had been suffering from 'a marvellous faint and feeble heart with intermittent fever' and on the day that he wrote he had 'fallen into a great sweat'.[4]

The birth of Princess Elizabeth restored the situation regarding the succession to where it had been before the annulment of the king's first marriage. He again had a legitimate daughter who would succeed to the crown and speculation that he would legitimise Henry Fitzroy was ended by the youth's death, in July 1536. The longed-for legitimate son had not been born, but the king had high hopes that his third wife, Jane Seymour, who he married in May 1536, would give birth to a boy. As he was growing into middle age, his anxieties about that vital aspect of his reign, leaving a legitimate son to succeed him, were increasing. When plague appeared in the summer of 1537, as the anticipated date of the birth of the queen's child grew steadily nearer, the king's and the queen's nervousness also intensified. On 21 July Lady Lisle was told that one of the gentlemen of Lady Rutland's household had died of the plague. Perhaps that was what so alarmed the queen: 'Your Ladyship would not believe how much the Queen is afraid of the sickness; yet the mortality is not so great as last year, for there died in London last week but 112'.[5] The figures for the numbers of deaths provided evidence of the scale of the danger, as they were meant to do, but did not reduce the concern. The response contrasted with that in 1533, for instead of the king and queen travelling around minimising the number of their contacts, Jane was ensconced at Hampton Court with very few companions and staff, while everyone else was kept away. In the past the monarch had been isolated by evading everybody except a few during epidemics, now everyone else was ordered to do the evading and stay away from the king and queen. Even Cromwell absented himself, working from St James's Palace.

On 12 October 1537, the queen gave birth to a boy, the future Edward VI. The king was delighted, of course, to have a son, but also to have a legitimate male heir at last, after so many years of hoping for one. In his eyes, this justified his actions, in having his first two marriages annulled, and in the major political measures that had been part of the process, essentially the English Reformation. He would have expected that his male heir would be seen to vindicate his actions in the courts of Europe, so that the birth was a diplomatic as well as a dynastic triumph. Immediately, though, it did pose the dilemma of whether to have a quiet christening with few people present, following the cautious arrangements of recent months, or to have a full celebration, with the aristocracy, senior clergy and diplomats present. It is not at all surprising that the king opted for the latter, and the prince was christened in the chapel at Hampton Court, where a congregation of 400 assembled, notwithstanding the continuing danger of plague. But two of the members of the nobility who had been chosen to carry the prince from his mother's chambers to the chapel decided that it would be unsafe for them to travel from Croydon Palace to Hampton Court, 13 miles away, because of the risk of transferring the infection. And the sheriffs of London were warned that they should restrict people from going from the city to the palace on the day of the christening 'on account of the plague'. The event went according to plan, the congregation was kept away from the royal party and the prince was returned to the queen's apartments before being moved to his own isolated rooms elsewhere in the palace. The queen had sickened after the birth and failed to recover, dying on 24 October. The sorrowful king left Hampton Court and as Edward began to grow up he was, in the words of his own journal, 'brought up, [un]til he came to six years old, among the women'.[6]

The prince's upbringing was mostly at Hampton Court, where the king had a self-contained range of buildings erected for the boy's household. Built across the north side of Chapel Court and isolated from the rest of the complex, this contained its own kitchen, as well as a bedchamber, watching-chamber and presence-chamber. It also had a bathroom and a garderobe. Creating the prince's establishment provided the opportunity to apply standards and regulations to a royal household which would protect its members from diseases. A set of instructions was issued in March 1539 controlling Edward's household, which was under the direction of Sir William Sidney, as Chamberlain of the household, and Sir John Cornwallis, as Steward.[7] Sidney had served the crown throughout Henry's reign, as soldier, sailor and officer of the household, with diplomatic assignments as well. His instructions were to oversee the prince's 'bread and meat, his raiment, and the control of persons resorting to him, the avoidance of infection, and the economic management of the household'. A whole raft of matters was mentioned, including the preparation of food and the tasting of it before it was served to the prince. Cleanliness was deemed important, for the walls, floors and even the ceilings of his lodgings were to be scrubbed several times each day, new clothes were to be washed, 'aired at the fire', brushed and perfumed before he wore them, and others were to try on his clothes before he did, in case they had been poisoned. An interesting rule was that those who attended the prince had to be of the knightly class or of higher status. That may have been to maintain the social status of his household at a senior level, that only those of such standing could be trusted, or perhaps because they were thought to be less susceptible to disease than the lower orders; that was a generally accepted characteristic of plague at the time.[8]

Obviously, anyone who showed symptoms of an illness was to be prevented from coming into the prince's presence. But that was too general a rule, and the instructions were quite specific in a clause which stated: 'to avoid all infection and danger of pestilence and contagious diseases that might chance or happen in the Prince's household by often resorting of the officers or servants of the same to London, or to some infected and contagious places, his Majesty's said servants shall provide and put such order as none of his grace's privy chamber, none of the officers as have any office about his grace's person, or in his household, shall resort to London, or to any other place, during the summer or contagious time'. Those who did so because they had tasks to carry out should not on their return go into the prince's presence or go near him for as many days as the Chamberlain or Steward should decide. If any person should suddenly fall sick, then at once he or she should be 'removed out of the house'. But the Instructions did not contain only those rules with respect to the prevention of disease. It also noted that the officers and servants, such as the cooks, yeomen and grooms of the hall, employed 'sundry boys, pages, and servants, which without any respect go to and from, and be not wary of the dangers of infection, and do often times resort into suspect places'; the king's order was that 'they shall be restrained from having any servant boy or page, and none to be admitted within the house'. To prevent the risk of contracting infection transmitted by the poor people who came to the gate for alms, a place was to be established 'a good way from the gates' where they would collect their alms from the almoners and then leave. But if any beggar should 'presume to draw near the gates, then they may be appointed to be grievously punished, to the example of others'.[9]

The chance to design both the buildings, which were distant from a city and furthermore could be maintained separately from the complex in which they stood, as well as to control the daily operation of a royal household, was the ideal way to implement the policy of reducing the vulnerability of members of the royal family to disease. Plague and the sweating sickness were doubtless regarded as the most threatening; the most recent outbreak of the sweat had occurred less than six years before the prince's household was established. But others were also dangerous and, to the king's horror, in the autumn of 1541 Edward contracted malaria while at Hampton Court; it was described as 'a quartan fever' and was said to be unusual for a child of his age who was 'not of a melancholic complexion'. After receiving the news the king became so anxious that he summoned his most favoured physician, Dr William Butts, to attend the prince, and also 'all the doctors in the country'.[10] The prince survived, but that alarm showed that even the best practices of cleanliness and control of access were not guaranteed to keep sicknesses away; the isolation policy had not worked. Nevertheless, it was retained when plague struck again in 1543, prompting a renewal of the regulations, including proclamations ordering that nobody from London should so much as enter the gates of any house where the king and queen were present, nor should anyone go from the court to London and then return. Those who had had plague in their house or visited anyone infected, or even lived near a place where the plague was then present, or had recently been, should not go to court or allow any attendants of the court to enter their houses.[11] Those orders were not put to the ultimate test because the sweating sickness did not strike again in Henry's reign and was not to reappear until after Edward had succeeded his father in January 1547, but it returned in 1551.

The first year of the new reign was marked by a plague outbreak in London, which lingered into the autumn. On 15 November the corporation ordered that all houses infected with the plague since the beginning of the month should be marked by a St Anthony's cross (a headless cross resembling the Greek letter tau), which was to remain for 40 days. It also required all the wells and pumps to have their water drawn on three days each week and at least 12 buckets of water should be washed down the channels in the streets, to clean them. Plague claimed victims in the city again in the following year, with the law courts adjourned on 28 August.[12]

Edward maintained the same medical establishment as his father had done, which consisted of three physicians, six surgeons and three apothecaries.[13] It may have been that the council acted on the advice of the doctors, or perhaps of that of the aldermen, when it abruptly moved the king to Hampton Court on 11 July 1551. That was barely in time, for in his journal the king had already noted 'came the sweat into London', referring to the 9th or 10th of the month. The Chronicle of the Grey Friars put the date of its appearance at 9 July, but the parish register of St Dionis Backchurch recorded the burial of a person who died 'of the sweat' on the 5th. Edward VI's figure for the number of deaths on 10 July was 70, and 120 on the 11th. He described it as 'more vehement than the old sweat' and a gentleman of his household and one of his grooms died of the disease. Dr John Caius later wrote that it reached London three days earlier, on 7 July. He tracked its progress from Shrewsbury in the middle of April, from where it advanced 'with great mortality to Ludlow, Presteigne, and other places in Wales, then to Chester, Coventry, Oxford, and other towns in the south, and such as were in and about the way to London'. The named places must have been where Caius had informants, and many other places must have experienced the disease before it reached the capital, where he described it as 'there continuing sore'. Henry Machyn noted in his diary that the disease erupted in London on 7 July and it caused the deaths of 'many merchants and great rich men and women, young men and old, of the new sweat'. Use of the words 'old' and 'new' may have indicated awareness from its symptoms of a variation in the strain of the virus, or perhaps it meant a fresh outbreak of the disease which had been dormant for 18 years.

According to the Venetian envoy, the effect in London was depressing: 'The alarm ... was great and universal, especially at the courts, some of the King's chamber attendants having died, so that his Majesty and all who could made their escape, all business being suspended, the shops closed, and nothing attended to, but the preservation of life'. John Stow wrote that it was 'a terrible time in London, for many a one lost suddenly his friends, by the sweat'. Stow also believed that 'the people being in the best health were suddenly taken', partly due, in his opinion, to the lack of proper nursing at the outset, so that some died within 12 hours of contracting the disease. He cited the case of seven householders who supped together and before eight o'clock the following morning six of them had died. After it had ended in London 'it went from thence through all the east parts of England into the north until the end of August, at which time it diminished, and in the end of September fully ceased'. The care with which the sweat was tracked across England was matched by the records made of the number of its victims in London. Although the record of those who died of the disease on 7 and 8 July was not kept, from 9 July until the 16th it claimed 761 victims, and a further 143 between then and 30 July. That was a total of 904 deaths in 21 days, 761 of them in the first seven days, which suggests that the king noted the figure for 11 July because that was the worst day.[14] Machyn's figure was 872 deaths from all causes between 8 and 19 July, while another record covering 7 July until 20 July gave 938, plus an unknown number of others down to 23 July. In the registers of 28 City parishes, 90 per cent of burials were recorded in the eleven days between 10 and 20 July. Within the City, three deaths from the sickness were registered at St Dionis, Backchurch, and eleven in the register of St Antholin, Budge Row, with the note: 'In the time of the sweating July', 1551. Beyond the City, just two burials in St Martin-in-the-Fields were annotated 'ex sudore' (from the sweat); there could have been more that were not identified and that parish may have escaped relatively lightly. A letter written on 2 August by one Christopher Froschover gives the number of dead in London as 2,000.[15] The City's population was roughly 80,000 and that of the metropolis was approximately 150,000.

While Caius's information on the chronology and death toll was good, his account of the geographical spread of the disease was inadequate. He may have been in Shrewsbury that spring and observed the disease there, but the town's chronicle gave the beginning of the epidemic as 22 March, rather than Caius's mid-April. John Stow also gave Shrewsbury as the place of origin of the epidemic and 15 April as the date when it was identified and wrote that it subsided in the north of England at the end of September. Caius may have been his source. It is likely that the disease first appeared, or was recognised, in late March onwards in the Welsh borders, and perhaps also in Devon and Lancashire, and erupted across the Midlands in the following months. It was identified at Loughborough on 24 June. Special penitentiary church services were ordered and, for the first time in the Church of England's short existence, in June a new liturgy was devised and issued for them. The practice was followed in later disasters.[16]

Parish registers had not yet been compiled during earlier outbreaks and so they provide a new tool for identifying the areas to which the disease spread, with the proviso that the burial entries recorded the reading of the burial service, not the interments themselves. That may have allowed some under-recording if, for example, the parish clerk and the clergy were themselves victims or were overwhelmed by the numbers of bodies to be disposed of and so no services were held. No records were maintained of the victims who fell seriously ill with the sweating sickness, or any other disease, but who survived. Places which suffered for a time from the effects of the sweat may not have left a record of the outbreak. At Worcester, parish registers which have survived show higher than average mortality for the years 1545 and 1558, but not for 1551, when the sweating sickness hit the region and presumably the city as well. Chester experienced high numbers of deaths in 1537, 1550 and 1556, all attributed to 'plague', yet there is separate evidence to show that the city was hit by the sweating sickness in 1551.[17]

Despite the limitations of the evidence, the characteristics of the disease in 1551 can be broadly identified. In almost one-third of 680 parish registers that have survived, with a wide national spread, there is some evidence that the sweat struck the community. That was commonly in a single burst of just a few days, for the disease did not linger. At Marbury in Cheshire, nine of the thirteen burials marked in the register as dying from the sweating sickness were carried out between 14 and 17 July, and in Darley, Derbyshire, nine burials of victims of the sickness were interred between 5 and 10 July. In Devon, at East Down, there were twelve burials between 15 and 22 August, with five on a single day, and at Uffculme 27 interments were carried out between 2 and 11 August, with a peak on the 5th and the 6th. In eastern England, the same feature can be identified, with 11 deaths in Thaxted in Essex, specified as being from the sweat, in four days in July. At Chelmsford and Terling, both in the same county, the pattern was rather different, with two bursts of burials of victims, separated by a break, suggesting two separate sources of infection. Overall, the death rate in July was 105 per cent above the current average and in August it was 34 per cent.[18] Such a burst of high mortality was severe enough to make an impact on communities across England without being sustained enough to affect the country's population size or trends.

The registers confirm Caius's description of the extent of the disease, with beginnings in the Shropshire, Herefordshire and Worcestershire region, erupting from there during June and affecting especially Cheshire, Staffordshire and Warwickshire, *en route* to London. At Chester, the mayor, Edmund Gee, was said to have attended a meeting of a local court in the morning and died before that evening, and the city's death toll was reported to have been 40 victims within 24 hours.[19] Bristol was hit by early July, when the parish of St Nicholas saw a rise in burials; the other central city parishes, for which there are no comparable records, probably suffered the same experience. They then endured, in 1552, what probably was a plague outbreak, with a rise in burials in the late summer and autumn months; over the whole year, they were more than five times the normal level. It was said that in 1551-2 there was 'the greatest mortality by pestilence in Bristol that any man knew'.[20] The city was the third largest in England, after London and Norwich, with a population of more than 10,000, so a sweating sickness epidemic would have had a considerable impact, there and in the surrounding area.

The south-east of England was infected after London, with Croydon afflicted in early July and burials in Kent, Essex (where seven of the 32 parishes for which register evidence survives experienced deaths from the disease), Suffolk and Cambridgeshire, and the north in late July and August, through until September. Froschover's letter puts the death toll in Cambridge at 200.[21] Durham was reached by 21 July and Lancashire during late July and August. In Yorkshire, an outbreak of plague also occurred and the officials in York recorded in October the presence of disease 'now perceived to be a kind of plague and sweating'. The city and Hull both suffered in the outbreak. The disease generally withered away at the end of September, although a few places experienced it during the autumn, such as Louth in Lincolnshire in October and Rye in Sussex in November and December. A feature of the epidemic which is shown by the register analysis is that the malady struck rural parishes as well as the towns and cities; it was not predominantly an urban disease and villages could experience a high intensity of mortality. It also shows that contemporary descriptions of it carrying off more males than females probably were correct, but with the differential being higher in towns than in the countryside, and that the wealthy suffered high mortality, as well as the poor. Comments concerning the relative immunity of children in any of the sweating sickness outbreaks cannot be verified. One contemporary comment was that 'few aged men, or women and children, died thereof'.[22]

Young adult males were regarded as being especially susceptible, reflected in local descriptions. At Loughborough, the parish register described it as the 'sweat called *New acquaintance*, alias *Stoop Knave and know thy master*'. In the Devon parish of Uffculme it was called 'The hot sickness called Stopgallant'. Thomas Hancock wrote in his autobiography that 'God plagued this realm most justly for our sin with three notable plagues'. One of them he designated the 'posting sweat, that posted from town to town through England, and was named *stop gallant,* for it spared none, for they were dancing in the court at 9 o'clock that were dead by eleven o'clock'. John Jones, in 1566, also described it as 'a sweat called stoupegalante'.[23] Those comments imply that it struck down young, self-confident men in their prime, a description that would certainly have applied to Henry and Charles Brandon, sons of Charles Brandon, Duke of Suffolk and long-term friend, and brother-in-law, of Henry VIII. They had enrolled at St John's College, Cambridge, in 1549 and after the sweating sickness had reached the town they moved to Buckden in Huntingdonshire, where the Bishop of Lincoln's palace offered a possible refuge. But they both died of the disease there, within half an hour of each other, on 14 July. They were 14 and 16 years old and their deaths brought the male line to an end and the loss of the dukedom and the other family titles.[24]

News of the Brandons' deaths would have sent a shudder through the royal household and dismayed those responsible for the safety of members of the aristocracy and other senior figures during such a dangerous sickness. They had, after all, been following the practice commonly pursued in such hazardous times. For the policy of isolation to be effective, those who were to be protected required good information and judgement and sound and timely advice, which the Brandons clearly did not have. They should have left Cambridge earlier, set out for separate destinations and certainly should not have travelled together. Buckden probably was chosen as a refuge because it was large enough to entertain such senior figures; Katherine of Aragon had been sent there by Henry VIII in 1533 and the king and his new wife, Catherine Howard, had stayed there in 1541. Henry Holbeach had officiated at the funeral of the Duke of Suffolk in 1545 and been appointed Bishop of Lincoln two years later; clearly he was favoured by the family and his position as bishop may have been a factor in the choice of his palace as the brothers' refuge. But Buckden was a thoroughfare village, not at all secluded, on the Great North Road and standing alongside the navigable River Ouse. Its advantages for the Brandons' stay were offset by its disadvantages, and of course, the youths could have contracted the disease before they left Cambridge. Bishop Holbeach was also said to have died of the sweating sickness, three weeks after the Brandons, in early August 1551, at Nettleham, close to Lincoln.

The Brandons' fate could have been that of any family which acted without due caution; it could even have happened to the Tudors and their deaths do explain to some extent Henry VIII's great concern with the sweating sickness. The boys' grandfather had been killed at Bosworth, fighting for Henry Tudor, their uncles had played an important role in Henry's reign and their father had been a key figure at Henry VIII's court, marrying Henry's sister Mary. Sir Henry Brandon had continued to play the kind of role at Edward VI's court upon which his father's career had been built and he was very much in the king's favour. Yet that social and political advancement which was the ambition of members of the sixteenth-century nobility, bringing power and prestige, were wiped out within a few hours, possibly within an hour. The deaths naturally attracted attention and the youths drew the praise often given to those who die young. Caius referred to them as examples of 'such persons so notably noble in birth, goodly conditions, grave sobriety, singular wisdom, and great learning, as Henry Duke of Suffolk, and the lord Charles his brother, as few hath been seen like of their age'.[25] Such approval was scant consolation for such a serious misjudgement when faced with a threat that had been around for more than 60 years.

The Swiss theologian Josua Maler, who was in his early twenties, toured parts of southern England with a friend in 1551. They travelled to Gloucester, where they arrived on 30 June and after meeting John Hooper, Bishop of Gloucester, in the Cotswolds they returned to Oxford. Despite the sweating sickness being prevalent in that part of the Midlands, they left Oxford on 7 August to go to London, showing no sense of urgency to get away from the danger and breaking their journey for sight-seeing at Syon House, Brentford and Richmond, 'where a large number of the King's councillors were accommodated'. They went on to Hampton Court, but of course could not gain an audience with the king, who was closeted there for his safety. Nor were they in a hurry to leave London having arrived in the city and taken time to see its sights before taking a ship to Vlissingen on 15 August. In his journal, Maler made no mention of being aware of the disease and the risks he and his friend were running, and their insouciance was justified, for they got away without being infected. He suggests an altogether different impression of how things were in London and southern England during the height of the epidemic than the nervous anxiety conveyed by Machyn and Stow, both of whom were Londoners.[26]

The king showed an interest in the decline of the disease and on 24 September 1552 wrote from Windsor to his friend Barnaby FitzPatrick, summoning him back to court with the reassurance that 'for sickness,

I hear of no place where any sweat or plague has reigned, but only in Bristol, and in the country near about. Some suspected it to be among a few in the town of Poole in Dorsetshire, but I rather think not. For I was within three mile of it and less, and yet no man feared it'.[27] The total number of deaths from the sweating sickness in the epidemic was roughly 15,000, from a population in England and Wales of roughly three million, although of course in some places the proportion was much higher than these figures suggest.

Like plague, the sweating sickness was deployed by religious writers and others as a call to repent and live a more religious life when the epidemic had subsided. These were not always formal or futile entreaties. A generation after the sweating sickness of 1551 the chronicler Raphael Holinshed wrote that it had 'enforced the people greatly to call upon God, and to do many deeds of charity'.[28] At the height of the epidemic, on 18 July, the king sent a circular letter to the bishops because he was 'vexed with this extreme and sudden plague that daily increased over all'. This was attributed to:

> the peoples' wickedness through the which the wrath of god hath been thus marvellously provoked, for the more we study how to instruct them in the knowledge of god, and of his most holy word that consequently they might follow and observe his laws and precepts: so much the more busy is the wicked spirit to alienate their hearts from all godliness and his malice hath so much prevailed that because the people are become as it were open rebels against the divine God.

He had sent one plague after another and now 'he hath thrown forth this most extreme plague of sudden death'. To assuage His wrath, the bishops were, through the ministers in their dioceses, to 'persuade the people to resort more diligently to common prayer then they have done and there not only to pray with all their hearts in the fear of god as good and faithful men should do' but also to persuade their parishioners to amend their lifestyles and specifically 'to refrain their greedy appetites from that insatiable serpent of covetousness where with most men are so infected that it seems each one would devour another without charity or any godly respect to the poor to their neighbours or to their common wealth for the which god hath not only now poured out this plague upon them'. The ministers themselves were partly to blame for the catastrophe, having been 'both so dull and so feeble in discharging of their duties that it is no marvel though their flocks wander, not knowing the voice of their shepherd and much less the voice of their principal and sovereign master'.[29]

Covetousness and greed were obvious targets for the church, which for centuries had preached the virtues of abstinence and self-restraint. Fasting was part of the church's annual pattern, not only during the 40 days of Lent leading up to Easter but on other days in its calendar. Yet indulgence had become more common among the laity, offsetting, as the church's hierarchy saw it, the good produced by prayer and fasting. It also diminished the church's authority by ignoring its teachings as individuals attempted to enhance their social standing through the quality and quantity of the foods and drink served, the fineness of the cuisine, the richness of the plate and vessels in which they were served, and the splendour of decorations in the rooms where they were enjoyed. As the Protestant reformers gained ground over the Catholic traditionalists in the early years of Edward's reign, the sickness provided an opportunity to reiterate the church's disapproval of indulgence and excess. That extended to clothing, décor and personal adornments. It had been common since the Black Death to condemn sinfulness as a cause of an epidemic; blaming extravagance while not mentioning some of the common failings of humanity was a more up-to-date take on the causes of epidemic disease. It was in that context that the contents of the king's letter should be seen, taking the opportunity of reiterating the point about excess and extending it beyond the well-to-do specified in the sumptuary legislation, apparently to all members of the church's congregations.

The bishops began to discuss a revision of the Book of Common Prayer in January 1551 and it was issued in the following year. They were, therefore, considering its contents when the epidemic of sweating sickness occurred. Whether because of that outbreak, or the continuing affliction of plague, influenza and other diseases, it contained a supplication to the Almighty to 'have pity upon us miserable sinners, that now are visited with great sickness and mortality, that like as thou did then [in the time of King David] command thy angel to cease from punishing: So it may now please thee to withdraw from us this plague and grievous sickness, through Jesus Christ our Lord'. The Polish theologian Jan Laski and his wife were in England and Archbishop Cranmer offered them a refuge at the archbishop's palace in Croydon when the epidemic struck. Unfortunately, his generosity backfired and they both contracted the disease, as did Cranmer's physician John Herd. Mrs Laski died in the following year; Jan and Herd both survived but had to endure a period of convalescence and Jan suffered from severe headaches thereafter.[30]

In 1553 Bishop Hooper issued *An Homily to be read in the time of pestilence*, in which he stated that 'sin and the transgression of God's law is the very cause and chief occasion of pestilence and of all other diseases', and that superstition and false religion, and an ignorant or negligent clergy, were the causes of pestilence. To punish those offences, God 'so alters, not by chance, nor by the influence of stars, the wholesomeness of the air into pestilent and contagious infection'. These represented the reactions of the clergy in the aftermath of the sweating sickness outbreak and the continued threat of plague.[31] Bishop Hooper had been directly affected by the epidemic, as he wrote on 1 August 1551: 'my wife, and five others of my chaplains and domestics, were attacked by a new kind of sweating sickness, and were in great danger for twenty-four hours. I myself have but recently recovered from the same. The infection of this disease is in England most severe'.[32] Like Machyn, Hooper referred to the malady as 'new'.

The sweating sickness ushered in a decade of high mortality. In 1554 the Venetian envoy Giacomo Soranzo wrote that there was 'some little plague in England well nigh every year, for which they are not accustomed to make sanitary provisions, as it does not usually make great progress; the cases for the most part occur amongst the lower classes, as if their dissolute mode of life impaired their constitutions'.[33] That was not entirely accurate so far as putting counter-measures in place was concerned, but does convey the almost routine increases in the numbers of deaths, especially during the summer and autumn months. Further heavy mortality came with an outbreak of influenza across the country in the late 1550s and the mid-century period culminated in a plague epidemic in 1563 which was the deadliest outbreak of the century. People must have waited with trepidation for the next epidemic to strike, as it was not yet apparent that the sweating sickness had ceased to be a major killer and would not return with one of its characteristic short and sharp outbreaks. Raphael Holinshed's *Chronicles*, published in 1557, described the disease as 'so sharp and deadly that the like was never heard of to any man's remembrance before that time'.[34]

Those who experienced a fever with what seemed to be the attributes of the sweating sickness were inclined to diagnose their malady as being a case of the disease. John Jones was at Lord St John's house at Southampton in 1558 when he contracted a fever that he equated with the sweat that had caused the epidemic in 1551. It had a debilitating effect on him, for 'notwithstanding the great sweat, it was long after before I recovered of my health, so that the said sweat did nothing profit'.[35] As a writer on the subject, Jones should have correctly diagnosed the disease, and if he did so then he was the victim of one of its last occurrences in England, but not quite the final one.

Chapter Eight

Recollections

The last three Tudor monarchs did not have children and so the specially arranged apartments at Hampton Court and the household orders of 1539 were not developed further. They had been a dead end so far as controlling epidemic disease was concerned, although of course that could not have been known at the time and the principles of isolation and controlled movement had been firmly established. Elizabeth followed her father's example in going on royal progresses during the summer months, showing herself to her subjects in south-east and southern England and the Midlands, thereby adding to the aura of monarchy and encouraging a sense of loyalty. Even though most of her progresses were arranged in advance and involved sometimes short stays at the houses of her subjects, rather than her own, some were prompted by an imminent risk of disease. After the great epidemic in 1563-4, the country experienced no major plague outbreaks until those in 1593-4, although the intervening years were peppered with eruptions of the disease, many regional rather than national in extent. In 1593 the queen and the court were said to 'keep in out places, a great part of the household being cut off from London' because of the plague.[1]

The sweating sickness was not said to have contributed to the public health crises during Elizabeth's reign. When Nicholas Faunt mentioned its presence in London in 1583, more than 30 years had passed since the epidemic of sweating sickness in 1551. He had been educated at Gonville and Caius College and then Corpus Christi College in Cambridge, graduating from Corpus in 1576. Within two years, in 1578 he had become secretary to Sir Francis Walsingham, who supervised the government's intelligence gathering. Faunt came to know Anthony

Bacon of Gorhambury, Hertfordshire, eldest son of Sir Nicholas Bacon and brother of Francis, who had also been educated at Cambridge, and they were then rising in the world. Anthony and Faunt became close friends as well as collectors of information for Walsingham. Faunt was familiar with Paris and was there when Anthony obtained a licence to travel abroad, going first to Geneva and then to Paris, before making journeys across France. Faunt, meanwhile, had been recalled by Walsingham and he kept in touch with Anthony by letters, summarising the situation in England. Anthony occasionally failed to respond quickly, because of the ill-health that had troubled him since he was at Cambridge and persisted thereafter. He complained so much of his problems that some of his acquaintances suspected that what he was really suffering from was hypochondria and of taking too much of the readily available 'physic' concocted from herbs.[2]

In a letter of 6 May 1583 Faunt told Anthony about the state of public health in London and the prospects for the coming summer.[3] He was not optimistic, predicting that 'there would be a great mortality in the approaching summer, since the infection was already very great both in the city and the country, especially in all great towns throughout the kingdom'. He went on to write that he 'heard of certainty, that the sweating sickness was on foot in London, or some such like contagious and pestiferous disease; but of hot fevers, that were little better, all the world complained already; so that her majesty would not reside long so near London, and the next term, it was thought, would not be held in any place'. As an indication of how disruptive the outbreaks had been he mentioned that Parliament 'which had been so often prorogued, and had so many sessions, was now wholly broken up; so that it was not likely, that there should be any for a good while'. Someone of Faunt's experience in gathering and summarising information was hardly likely to make a mistake when referring to a disease as the sweating sickness, although the reference is slightly weakened by his use of the term 'some such like contagious and pestiferous disease' and mention of 'hot fevers'. Even after an interval of 30 years, the identification of the sweat should have been secure, but there is no corroborative evidence; if it did not cause a death which was described as being from the disease, then no formal record would have been created.

But consciousness of the disease remained, even after its impact had become less immediate. The term 'burning fever' was adopted by John Florio in his translation of Michel de Montaigne's *Essays*. The author wrote about accidents and unforeseen circumstances which could kill someone suddenly, and the good or ill fortune, and pure chance, that might lead to premature death. Montaigne published his *Essays* in 1580 and Florio, in his English translation issued in 1603, put the writer in the position of musing on 'someone or other, that but few days before was taken with a burning fever, and of his sudden end, coming from such a feast or meeting where I was myself, and with his head full of idle conceits, of love, and merry glee; supposing the same, either sickness or end, to be as near me as him'. The writer had been fortunate and had a lucky escape in not contracting the disease to which his acquaintance had succumbed. Montaigne never came to England and although he should have known of the sweating sickness by repute he would have had no direct knowledge of it, while Florio would have been aware of its characteristics; the 'burning fever' producing a sudden death does suggest that he was implying that the sweat was what had struck down the victim.[4]

Faunt also told Anthony, by way of reassurance, that 'many devices and orders were already set forth for the avoiding of these dangerous diseases'. On 21 April the Privy Council, anxious about the possibility of a plague outbreak, had written to the Lord Mayor and aldermen to make the point 'that they should see that all infected houses were shut up, and provision made to feed and maintain the sick persons therein, and for preventing their going abroad; that all infected houses were marked, the streets thoroughly cleaned, and a sufficient number of discreet persons appointed to see the same done'.[6] Those measures were the core of what had become government policy since the great plague epidemic of 1563. The response, in a reply written on the same day that Faunt wrote to Anthony Bacon, was that 'the Court of Aldermen had published certain orders, which they intended to execute with diligence', and to complain that leisure activities beyond the corporation's jurisdiction and control were contributing to the problem. These were summarised as 'the assemblies of people to plays, bear-baiting, fencers, and profane spectacles at the Theatre and Curtain and other like places, to which great multitudes of the worst sort of people resorted'.[5] The Theatre and Curtain were two playhouses to the north of the City, in Shoreditch, which were attracting the corporation's attention; the Theatre was erected in 1576, and the Curtain was built close by in the following year. Faunt would have read the correspondence and that might have prompted him to include the topic of public health in his letter to Anthony, although it would have been high on the agenda in any case. The first plague orders for London were issued during that month, after several years of discussion as to the best course to be adopted. But the City had not built a pesthouse to which the sick could be moved for isolation once their symptoms had been diagnosed. The Privy Council reprimanded the aldermen and tried to embarrass them with the observation that 'other cities of less antiquity, fame, wealth, and reputation had provided themselves with such places whereby the lives of the inhabitants had been in all times of infection chiefly preserved'. The City was goaded by this to order, in May 1583, a survey of a potential site for a pesthouse on the road between London and Canonbury.[7] But the enthusiasm and conviction that the practice would work were still missing and the building was not erected for another ten years.

In the aftermath of the outbreak in 1563 the corporation's policy had been clearly stated. It ordered that 'blue headless crosses' (St Anthony crosses) should be attached to infected houses, the streets were to be regularly cleaned and bedding from infected houses should be burned. Household quarantine was to be enforced, with those in an infected house remaining there for a month and anyone who went out to buy provisions should carry a white rod two feet long so that others could give them a wide berth. Fires were to be lit in the streets on three evenings each week, to circulate stagnant air, and stray dogs, who were suspected of carrying the corrupt air and infection, were to be killed by the dog catcher. The problem of the number of poor who could not obtain work because of the disrupted economy was dealt with by an order that the parishes should take a special collection for the poor. To avoid increasing the numbers of paupers, landlords were not to take tenants into houses or rooms left empty because their occupants had died of plague, and the constables were to search the alleys and lanes and send lists of such houses to the Lord Mayor. No householder was to take in anyone who had not been living in London for the previous three months, to deter those who were looking for a refuge in the city as local economies were disrupted. Plays and interludes were performed at inns and audiences crowding together risked the spread of the plague, and so they could be performed only after a licence had been obtained from the Lord Mayor.

The length of the period of quarantine, and hence the amount of support needed to maintain the poor, was debated by the corporation and the Council. In 1570 it was reduced to 20 days. In 1574 orders were issued that the words 'The Lord have mercy upon us' should be fixed to infected houses and that two people should be appointed in each parish to examine the body of anyone suspected to have died of plague, to decide if it really had been the cause of death. Two more women were to take provisions to those who were being held in quarantine, making it unnecessary for anyone from those houses to go out. The Council kept a sceptical eye on the enforcement of the measures, questioning the accuracy of the weekly returns of the numbers of victims and wondering if the orders were being properly enforced. William Cecil, Lord Burghley complained to the Lord Mayor of his neglect in not enforcing them, to which the response was to draw attention to the scale of the problem in such a populous city and the failings of the parish officers, who naturally feared for their safety in pursuing their enquiries in the areas where plague was present and the inhabitants were antagonistic, and if they were persistent and contracted the disease they might pass it on to their superiors.

The Council was aware of developments on the continent and following the severe plague epidemic in Italy in 1576 it obtained copies of the orders issued in Milan during the crisis.[8] A draft set of regulations to be executed 'throughout the realm' was then prepared in

1578 and revised after the College of Physicians had been consulted; it was then issued as a printed set of orders. London was exempt, after a consultation; the corporation was especially doubtful whether the orders could be enforced in the city, which required the levy of a weekly tax to support the victims, and that lists should be compiled of houses in multiple occupancy and of the inhabitants, effectively a local census, to be checked weekly to avoid clandestine burials. It also preferred its existing system of aldermen and parish officers to paid officials to administer the arrangements.

Those doubts had been overcome by May 1583 when the corporation's common council entered a set of plague orders applicable to the City in its journal. Printed orders were issued in the same month and reissued when the next epidemic struck in 1593.[9] The 21 clauses codified existing practices. The quarantine period was set at 28 days and half a dozen of the orders dealt with household quarantine and the maintenance of those who were affected; someone defying the rules by going around the streets while suffering with a plague sore was liable to a spell of 28 days in prison. A similar number of orders repeated measures concerning the maintenance and cleanliness of the streets and highways, and supervision of that work. Regulations for the disposal of the dead banned the attendance of children at interments and prohibited gatherings of people after a funeral; plays and interludes required a licence; stray dogs were to be killed; someone leaving the city was allowed to go but not to return within 28 days, which would reduce the size of the problem of indigent poor in the city while moving it on to the communities nearby. The problem of lodgers, or 'inmates', who had no connection with the household with whom they were staying, either familial or economic, had prompted an order in the previous year and was to become a major concern for both the national and civic governments. That was because they were thought to live in nasty and overcrowded conditions and that 'filthy keeping of their houses and of noisome and ill savours in the streets is one of the greatest occasions of the infection of the plague'.[10] As the city's population expanded rapidly and the government attempted to curb the process by prohibiting new building, pressure on space increased and the inmates came to be seen as a major problem in spreading plague.

The orders were issued towards the end of a period during which plague had struck fairly frequently. The Michaelmas Law term was adjourned from Westminster every year between 1574 and 1582, with the sole exception of 1580. Even in 1580, there were 128 plague deaths, with probably more than 1,000 in 1581, and in 1582 plague caused 2,976 of the 6,762 recorded deaths in London. Somewhat ironically, and despite Faunt's apprehensions, 1583 was not a particularly sickly year. Although the regulations were prompted by the threat of plague and became known as the plague orders, the measures were applicable to public health generally, including the risk of the sweating sickness. It may be that Faunt's mention of that disease in London, which would have been noticed by Walsingham, did encourage the Council and corporation to come to the point at last and issue the orders in May 1583. Faunt and Walsingham were in the business of collecting and presenting hard intelligence and issues such as epidemic diseases were within their brief. It is possible that the early 1580s, well within living memory of the 1551 outbreak, rather than the mid-1560s, were the last time that the sweating sickness was identified in England.

Anthony Bacon died in 1601 while Francis continued to prosper. Knighted in 1603, he was appointed Solicitor General in 1607, Attorney General in 1613, a privy councillor in 1616, Lord Keeper in 1617 and Lord Chancellor in 1618, when he was raised to the peerage as Baron Verulam. After being created Viscount St Albans in January 1621, his political career ended abruptly in the following May, when he was deprived of his offices. He had simultaneously pursued a scholarly career which generated a range of writings. Perhaps his fall from favour allowed him more time to complete some of his outstanding works; in 1622 he published a history of the reign of Henry VII. It included a description of the onset of the sweating sickness in 1485, for which Bacon had a number of descriptions to draw upon, in particular those of Polydor Vergil and John Caius. The most authoritative, or at least highly regarded, at the time was Caius's account of the epidemic in 1551, which dealt with what had by then become an historic rather than a threatening disease. Caius also had considerable standing for his role in the re-founding of Gonville Hall at Cambridge, as Gonville and Caius College, and reforms of the College of Physicians.

Raphael Holinshed also had Caius's work available to him. From the perspective of the 1570s, he described the successive outbreaks of sweating sickness within the chronological arrangement of his narrative of English history. The work was to have been part of a large compendium of current knowledge, historical and geographical, with England as its focus. The larger project did not come to fruition, but Holinshed was authorised to prepare and publish a narrative of British history, with contributions from other scholars. This appeared as a two-volume set in 1577 and despite its scale and cost it proved to be a commercial success. Shakespeare's generation would have turned to Holinshed for authoritative information on English history, down to their own times.[11]

Themes can be picked out of his chronological account, with the sweating sickness appearing in sections on 1485, 1505, 1518, 1528 and 1551. He not only reported the outbreaks but was formed an opinion, that a treatment devised during the first epidemic was effective and he averred that it had reduced the number of deaths during the disease's second onset: 'by the remedy found at the beginning of it [the sweating sickness], nothing like the number died thereof now this second time, as did at the first time until the said remedy was invented'. But by the time of the outbreak in 1518 its efficacy had been forgotten, which explained the high number of deaths, for 'it should seem that they little remembered, or at least neglected, the preservative remedy used in the first great sweating sickness in king Henry VII's time, whereby many a man's life was saved, so now the like benefit, by application of the same wholesome means, might have redounded to the patients'. But he believed that the treatment was revived in 1528. Briefly, 'the way to escape danger was close keeping moderately with some air and a little drink, and the same to be posset-ale, and so to keep them 30 hours, and then was the danger past; but beware of sudden cold'. Posset-ale was a bedtime drink of milk curdled with wine and spices. Despite the acceptance of a treatment for the disease, it was surely rather optimistic to claim that 'with lukewarm drink, temperate heat, and measurable clothes many escaped: few which used this order (after it was found out) died of that sweat'. Yet even by 1551, after more than 60 years of experience in nursing victims, according to Holinshed, the 'speedy riddance of life procured by this sickness, did so terrify people of all sorts, that such as could make shift, with money or friendship, changed their soil, and leaving places of concourse, betook them (for the time) to abodes, though not altogether solitary, yet less frequented'. He described Henry VIII's response in 1518, when the disease was prevalent from July to the middle of December, and in some places, a third, even a half, of the inhabitants died: 'the king kept himself ever with a small company, and held no solemn Christmas, willing to have no resort for fear of infection'. In a similar way, during the outbreak in 1528 the king 'for a space removed almost every day until he came to Tittenhanger, a place of the abbot of St Albans, and there he with the queen, and a small company about them, remained till the sickness was passed'. Holinshed's contemporaries probably accepted his descriptions as providing a rational description of the outbreaks, although some would have been surprised at the claims that he put forward for the success of the remedy which he described. The disease had indeed been 'a new kind of sickness' in 1485, killing most of those who were infected, including a 'great number' within London. The outbreak in 1528 had also produced a 'great mortality' and in 1551 men in their thirties, in particular, had succumbed. He supported the notion that the malady struck the English only, so that in Antwerp and other countries 'our Englishmen being there among divers other nations, only our Englishmen were sick thereof, and none other persons'.[12]

Devastating plague epidemics closely followed the accessions of James I in 1603 and his son Charles I in 1625. Four days after Charles came to the throne he ordered that rogues, vagabonds, beggars and prostitutes loitering at the gates of Whitehall Palace should be removed, reflecting his fastidious nature, as well as concern about the danger of contagion which dirty people were thought to represent.[13] The displacement of those regarded as posing a health risk was adopted by the Council as a means of protecting the royal household when plague threatened in 1636. Some Londoners sent their children to schools at Enfield, Waltham and other places close to the royal palace at Theobalds, and they or their servants visited them there, which was seen as a potential danger, and so the Council required that they should be removed. The numbers of houses held by Londoners in and around Kingston, Teddington and Isleworth were considered to increase the risk of plague infecting the nearby palaces of Hampton Court, Nonsuch and Oatlands. The Council responded by prohibiting anyone from travelling to them from the capital, at the risk of being removed from the houses or quarantined within them. In September it noted that refugees from the capital had brought the plague to Eltham, near the palace there, and it also ordered the evacuation of Londoners from houses within six miles of Windsor Castle.[14] The size of the areas specified and the potential numbers of people involved must have made implementation of those orders difficult, and had the regrettable effect of causing people to move at a time when there was a risk of transmitting disease. But the solution to the problem of protecting the royal family from plague now involved the quarantining or removal of people from considerable areas around a number of royal palaces, which was far removed from Henry VIII's response of skulking almost alone in the countryside for his own safety. He feared infection by the sweating sickness and the plague, but the Stuart monarchs had only to fear the plague, the sweating sickness having vanished.

The response to the major epidemic in 1665, the Great Plague, was less draconian. In fact, Charles II's court broke up in the summer as the scale of the outbreak became apparent, with the king going first to Syon House and then to Hampton Court, before moving on to Salisbury. When plague appeared in the city he transferred to Oxford, where Parliament assembled in October. Because the court went so far from the capital, on what resembled a royal progress more than a search for a sanctuary, regulations of the kind issued in 1636 to clear Londoners away from the vicinity of the nearby royal palaces were not necessary. The Great Plague was the last outbreak of the disease in Britain and so the need to protect the monarch from that infection also came to an end.

The disappearance of the sweating sickness towards the end of the sixteenth century was followed a century later by the end of the plague in northern Europe. Out of sight did not mean out of mind and anxieties about a resurgence of the plague occurred from time to time, especially when there were major epidemics in the Baltic lands and northern Germany in 1709-13 and in Provence in 1720-1. The government took appropriate countermeasures to prevent the disease coming into England, by quarantining shipping, and the fears were not realised. But other diseases caused alarm, such as a fever that Daniel Defoe, in 1712, claimed would precede a plague outbreak. The malady was attributed to soldiers returning from the War of the Spanish Succession. Not unnaturally, fear of plague far exceeded fear of the sweating sickness, which was altogether more remote and less threatening, and had not appeared elsewhere in Europe. Then there was a resurgence of interest in the sweat with the appearance in 1718 in a region of northern France of a fever that showed symptoms which bore some resemblance to those of the sweating sickness. Designated the Picardy Sweat, that malady recurred until 1861, but despite some similarities, it was not the same disease. In the autumn of 1721, the Privy Council considered the steps that should be taken if the plague reached London, although by then the epidemic in Provence was on the wane. Sir Hans Sloane, President of the College of Physicians, and his colleagues Richard Mead and John Arbuthnot were directed to investigate how the information recorded in the Bills of Mortality could be improved. Mead went on to prepare a book entitled *A Short Discourse concerning Pestilential Contagion and the Methods to be used to Prevent it*. In it, he repeated earlier proposals, especially those made by Sir Theodore de Mayerne in 1631 and the Earl of Craven in 1666, and he supported the policy of quarantining shipping from areas that were infected. He was convinced that contagion caused the spread of plague, but his views were controversial because the contagiousness of the disease was not universally accepted, and its incidence continued to be ascribed to local conditions and the effects of miasma. The debate between the contagionists and the anti-contagionists attracted considerable professional and lay attention and the debate continued through the eighteenth century and much of the nineteenth century, linked to the necessity of quarantining shipping, which was strongly opposed by many among the mercantile community.

Mead faced the difficulty encountered by all writers dealing with the plague and other epidemic diseases in the fifteenth and sixteenth centuries, which was how to classify the sweating sickness. It could not be omitted, for it had brought numerous deaths during its onslaughts, as had the plague itself, but it clearly had not been plague. Mead clearly struggled with the problem and wrote that it was 'not the common plague with glandular tumours, and carbuncles, yet a real pestilence from the same cause, only altered in its appearance, and abated in its violence, by the salutary influence of our climate'. To this he added that it shared many symptoms with plague, such as 'excessive faintness and inquietudes, inward burnings, &c. these symptoms being nowhere observed in so intense a degree as here they are described to have been, except in the true plague', and he regarded it as being a contagious disease, like the plague. He concluded that the sweating sickness was:

> a Plague with lessened Force: because though its carrying off thousands for want of right management was a proof of its malignity, which indeed in one respect exceeded that of the common plague itself (for few, who were destroyed with it, survived the seizure above one natural day) yet its going off safely with profuse sweats in twenty four Hours, when due care was taken to promote that evacuation, shewed it to be what a learned and wise historian calls it, rather a surprize to nature, than obstinate to remedies.

The fever in northern France in 1713, which he called the Dunkirk Fever, he described as 'the same kind of fever' and he attributed its origins to the plague in the Baltic, around Danzig.

Concern about the possibility of a plague outbreak continued through the eighteenth century, fuelled by epidemics in eastern Europe, while the sweating sickness became an ever more distant memory. That, and perhaps its popular name, allowed it to be treated with some levity and interest in it seems to have degenerated into the world of cartoons by the late eighteenth century. One such cartoon, after John Nixon, dated 1799, and entitled 'The Sweating Sickness' shows a corpulent figure of fun being taunted by his friends because he had the disease, and so missing his feast. (If he really did have the sweat, surely he would have been alone in the room?)[15]

General writers were able to draw upon the contemporary chronicles to provide as much information as their readers required. In his chapter on the reign of Henry VII in Volume 1 of his magisterial *The History of England*, David Hume mentioned the first onset of the disease, giving Polydore Vergil's account: 'There raged at that time in London, and other parts of the kingdom, a species of malady unknown to any other age or nation, the sweating sickness, which occasioned the sudden death of great multitudes ... In less than twenty-four hours the patient commonly died or recovered, but when the pestilence had exerted its fury for a few weeks, it was observed ... to be considerably abated.'

Medical and historical interest revived in the early nineteenth century. Some reasons for its having been remembered were put forward by Francis Webb, in 1857, in the terms of his own time, when he wrote that the disease was characterised by:

> the suddenness of its seizure, by its short and defined course of twenty-four hours, by its great fatality, by the profuse and fetid perspiration in which the patient was bathed, and from which the disease derived its most common name, by the frequency by which it attacked the same individual several times within a short period, or perhaps, we should more correctly say, by its relapsing tendency, by its selection of strong and robust men in the prime of life as its victims, by the equality with which it invaded the palaces of the rich and the cottages of the poor, we cannot wonder at its

producing a marked effect on the national mind, and being long held in remembrance.[16]

A professional approach to making sense of the chronology and typology of medieval and later diseases was adopted by the German scholars Christianus Gottfridus Grüner and J.C.D. Hecker. Grüner gathered extracts from contemporary sources for the disease in England and on the continent, which he issued as *Scriptores de sudore anglico superstites*, published in Jena in 1847. Hecker also became especially interested in the sweating sickness, issuing a separate publication on the disease that was translated into English in 1834 as *The Sweating Sickness: A medical contribution to the story of the fifteenth and sixteenth century*. Much of what was subsequently written about the disease was based on his work. J.S. Brewer, the editor of the monumental series the *Letters and Papers, Foreign and Domestic, Henry VIII*, a calendar of the state papers of the reign, did not shy away from dealing with the sweating sickness and included a section on the disease in volume 2, which covers the years 1515-1518. In it he printed an extract from Caius, but much more valuable were the mentions of the disease in the extracts included in the *Calendar*. He printed quotes from the papers in the Public Record Office (now The National Archives) to enliven what effectively was an essay on the sweating sickness during Henry VIII's reign. For example, in a letter to the Earl of Shrewsbury's chaplain Wolsey advised him to 'Tell your master, to get him into clean air, and divide his household in sundry places'. Brewer did not draw back from emphasising the horror of the disease:

> For centuries no infection had visited England, which in fearful rapidity and malignancy could be compared with the *sudor Anglicus*, as it was at first called, from the notion that its attacks were confined to Englishmen. People sitting at dinner, in the full enjoyment of health and spirits, were seized with it, and died before the next morning. An open window, accidental contact in the streets, children playing before the door, a beggar knocking at

the rich man's gate, might disseminate the infection, and a whole family would be decimated in a few hours without hope or remedy. Houses and villages were deserted. Where the sickness once appeared, precaution was unavailing; and flight afforded the only chance of security.

And he expressively summarised the mood around the court during the outbreaks of sweating sickness as one of 'general consternation and alarm'.

Caius's work remained the principal source for the disease and it was drawn upon by Charles Creighton in his *A History of Epidemics in Britain*, published in 1891. Creighton cast a critical eye over the evidence drawn upon for studies of the disease and especially the description in Caius, Hecker's hitherto widely respected source. Creighton complained of Hecker's reliance on Caius's 'gloomy rhetoric' and went so far as to claim that, aside from entries in parish registers, 'we have the generalities of Dr Caius, which amount to no more than a funereal essay, in the scholastic manner, upon the theme of sudden death. It may be doubted whether Caius really knew the facts about the disease in the country'. Creighton also attacked Hecker on the specific question of the first appearance of the sweating sickness in England, with the acerbic comment that he 'passed from the tradition of Polydore Virgil and of Caius, clean into the region of conjecture in assuming that the sweat had arisen among the French mercenaries on the voyage and on the march to Bosworth … There is nowhere a hint that it was prevalent among the troops, whether French, Welsh or English, who won the battle of Bosworth on the 22nd of August'.[17]

Caius identified the disease as a fever, producing pain 'in the back, or shoulder, pain in the extreme parts, as arm, or leg, with a flushing, or wind'; as well as 'grief in the liver and the near stomach. Thirdly, by the pain in the head, and madness of the same. Fourthly by the passion of the heart'. He accepted the framework of five epidemics, with their dates, already current and repeated since, although inflexibly, without the inclusion of other, less deadly or less well reported, outbreaks of the disease.¹⁸ With greater access to burial registers during the nineteenth and twentieth centuries, including the printing of many of them by local history societies, those occurrences should have become more apparent in the mid-sixteenth century. J.F.D. Shrewsbury's wide-ranging study of bubonic plague in the British Isles includes deaths from sweating sickness, although for 1551 he mentioned only London, Cambridge, Loughborough and Uffculme, and the two dukes of Suffolk at Buckden. Shrewsbury added nothing to the information on the incidence of the sweating sickness and it was to be a further 27 years before a more detailed investigation of burial records added to the available evidence.¹⁹

With the sole contemporary medical writer on the subject and his nineteenth-century interpreter thus disparaged, and no other medical or scientific evidence on which to draw, discussions on the nature and origin of the disease became more difficult. Those who wished to describe the nature of the disease and its relationship with plague fell back on Creighton's analysis, brought up to date by the consideration of later work with a scientific basis. Sir George Clark did attempt to rescue the reputation of Caius's account in his history of the Royal College of Physicians (1964), in which he urged that the two versions, in English and Latin, deserved praise for their originality 'for they give the first clinical descriptions of an epidemic disease by an Englishmen'. He also pointed out that Bacon had drawn upon them for his *History of Henry VII* 'and that is significant even if they do not point the way to effective epidemiology'. Indeed, in his study of epidemic diseases in fifteenth-century England, Robert Gottfried could offer no more than the comment that the sweating sickness was 'perhaps a form of influenza'. General writers on the period and those concentrating on specialities other than medical history have incorporated short accounts of the sweating sickness. Those have necessarily been without specialist knowledge and based on the contemporary accounts or studies deploying them. That category of authors included Mrs Henry Cust, in her book based on the journeys of four noblemen in the fifteenth and sixteenth centuries, which she published in 1909. One of the characters who came to her attention was Hubertus Thomas, who contracted and survived the sweat in 1529. As context, Mrs Cust included a brief account of the outbreak in that year and the recommended treatments of heating the patients and depriving them of liquids, which were the same in Germany as in England, and which she described as 'this rehearsal of hell'. Few writers have offered such a clear judgement or pithy condemnation of the care recommended for the victims as she did.[20]

The sweating sickness has attracted the attention of virologists and medical historians over the past 40 years or so, who have considered especially the nature of the disease, the means of transmission and its possible relationship with similar maladies. Scott and Duncan's description and analysis of the sweat in their much larger study of plague draws on published work of the twentieth century, giving considerable space to Creighton's account. They do not definitely support any of the suggestions but leave the reader with a summary of the state of knowledge, and speculation, when their book was published in 2001. The death and disruption caused by COVID-19 in 2020 prompted a renewal of the questions concerning the sweating sickness. But no conclusions can be drawn from the evidence.[21]

Contemporaries diagnosed the diseases that afflicted their communities and identified them by name, so that there was no confusion over attribution. Modern attempts to identify outbreaks of the sweating sickness in regions beyond England, the Calais area and those parts of the continent afflicted in 1529 are based on slender and unsupported evidence. The sweating sickness had not been confused by contemporaries with other maladies and certainly not with plague and several other diseases, including influenza, typhus and the pox. Creighton pointed out that the five major outbreaks were preceded by wet winters with heavy rainfall, suggesting that vermin leaving their burrows and finding shelter in houses and adjacent buildings could have helped to transmit the sweating sickness through their insect parasites. In that respect, the fact that the disease was not reported as spreading to upland Britain could be significant. If it was indeed a rodent-based disease, the black rat may have played a major role. Suggestions that the cause of the disease could have been a hemorrhagic fever or a hantavirus have received some support. Rodents, insects and bats act as carriers of the hantavirus family, which can cause severe respiratory illness, which would fit with the contemporary descriptions. But caution has been expressed regarding the notion of a hantavirus as the cause on the basis that it would have produced isolated cases across England; in fact, a detailed study of the 1551 outbreak and other, more scattered, evidence shows that such cases were in fact common, with a third of parishes suffering deaths from the disease. The author of the study of the epidemic in 1551 suggested arboviruses as the causative agent. Those possibilities are probably as close as virologists are likely to get to identifying the disease given the current state of knowledge. They do allow for a possible link with the Picardy sweat, despite the long interval between the outbreaks, while the disappearance of the sweating sickness is attributable to the spread of immunity among the English population.[22]

While medical information is sparse and the chroniclers of the Tudor period wrote from inconsistent information in terms of the groups which suffered worst and the levels of mortality, they do vividly convey the sense of urgent alarm and fear of the disease, and the pitiable reactions of those in communities, especially London, where it struck. In particular, the response of the king and the courtiers provides an insight into the reaction of the early Tudors to the sudden emergency that the disease represented. Short, sharp and deadly, an unidentified disease that attacked without warning unquestionably put genuine fear into the minds of Henry VIII and his people and for a time disrupted government, the law and the economy. The fear that it engendered could even frighten the credulous to death, according to Sir Brian Tuke.

Among the aspirations of a respectable citizen of Tudor England was to die a good death, peacefully in bed surrounded by relatives and friends, in the presence of a priest, having confessed his sins, made a will and settled any outstanding business and debts, and having asked forgiveness of those who might have taken offence in the past. The sweating sickness prevented that, with the ailing victim attended only by one or two hired nurses if they were fortunate, while everyone else had absented themselves, from the house as well as the room. According to Edward VI's notes on the disease, if a victim managed to obtain some respite with a few hours of sleep, when he awoke 'then he raved and should die raving', and did not pass calmly away.[23] By any standards, the sickness produced a bad death for its victims, who were left feeling abandoned, in excruciating pain, revoltingly smelly, disfigured by spots and dying in undignified circumstances that the individual would have wished to avoid, above almost all other things. Those who survived could suffer lifelong disorders, such as the painful headaches that afflicted Jan Laski, or, like John Colet, they could die of another cause after being weakened by the sweating sickness. Small wonder that the disease was long recalled with fear and loathing.

Appendix One

The Household Orders of 1539

These Orders were issued in 1539 to govern the management of the Prince of Wales's household at Hampton Court. They are taken from John Gough Nichols, *Literary Remains of King Edward the Sixth*, Roxburghe Club, I, 1857, pp. xxvii-xxx.

Instructions given by the king's highness unto his trusty and well beloved servants Sir William Sydney, Chamberlain of the household of the most noble and right excellent Prince Edward, Prince of Wales, Duke of Cornwall, Earl Palatine of Chester etc.; and to Sir John Cornwallis, Steward to his grace.

The king's highness wills that his said trusty and well beloved servants shall conceive in their minds that, like as there is nothing in the world so noble, just, and perfect, but that there is something contrary that evermore envies it, and procures the destruction of the same; insomuch, as God himself hath the devil repugnant unto him, Christ has his antichrists and persecutors, and from the highest to the lowest after such proportion, so the Prince's grace for all nobility and innocence (albeit he never offended any man), yet by all likelihood he lacks no envy or adversaries against his grace, who either for ambition of their own promotion, or otherwise for to fulfil their malicious perverse mind, would perchance, if they saw opportunity, which God forbid, procure to his grace displeasure; and although his excellent, wise, and prudent Majesty doubts not, but like as God for his consolation and comfort of all the whole realm has given the said Prince, so of his divine providence he will in the point of all danger preserve and defend him; yet, nevertheless, all diligent and honest heed, caution, and foresight ought to be taken to avoid (as much as man's wit may), all practices and evil enterprises, which might be devised against his grace, or the danger of his person; for, although almighty God is he that taketh cure and thought for us, and that he furnishes us of all necessaries, and defends us from all evils, yet his divine providence will have us to employ our diligences to the provision and defence of ourselves, and of such as be committed to our charge, as though it should not come of him, and that it notwithstanding we should know that without his helping hand our labour is futile, such is his bottomless divine providence.

Item, that the King's highness, for the special trust his grace hath conceived of his trusty servant Sir William Sydney, hath constituted him to be Chamberlain to the Prince's grace, and hath committed and appointed him as well to have the keeping, oversight, care, and cure of his Majesty and the whole realm's most precious jewel the Prince's grace, and foresee that all dangers and adversaries of malicious persons and casual harms (if any be) shall be vigilantly foreseen and avoided, as also such good order observed in his grace's household as may be to his majesty's honour, and assured surety of the Prince's grace person, our most noble and most precious jewel, for the which good order in the said household the said John Cornwallis being Steward together with the Vice-chamberlain and Comptroller, shall always join together.

Item, that for their best information, and for the first part of their instruction, they and every of them shall foresee that no manner stranger nor other person or persons, of what state, degree, dignity, or condition soever they be, except the Chamberlain, Steward, Vice-chamberlain, Comptroller, the lady Mistress, the Nurse, the Rocker, and such as be appointed continually to be in the Prince's grace privy chamber, and about his proper person, and officers in their offices, shall in any manner wise have access ordinary to touch his grace's person, cradle, or any thing belonging to his person, or have any entry or access into his grace's privy chamber, unless they shall have a special token or commandment express from the King's majesty, in the which case they shall regard the quality of the person, and yet nevertheless to suffer no such person to touch his grace, but only kiss his hand, and yet that no personage under the degree of knight to be admitted thereunto; and in this case the said Steward, Chamberlain, Vice-chamberlain, and Comptroller, or one of them at the least, to be ever present, and to see a reverent assay taken in due order ere [before] such person shall be admitted to kiss his grace's hand.

Item, that they shall at all times cause good, sufficient, and large assays of all kinds of bread, meat, and drinks, milk, eggs, and butter, prepared for his grace, and likewise of water, and of all other things that may touch his person or be ministered to him in any wise duly to be taken; to see his grace's linen, raiment, apparel whatsoever belonging to his person, to be purely washed, clean dried, kept, brushed, and reserved cleanly by the officers and persons appointed thereunto, without any intermeddling of other persons having no office there, in such wise as no danger may follow thereof; and before his grace shall wear any of the same, assays to be taken thereof as shall appertain, and that the Chamberlain and Vice-chamberlain, or one of them, shall daily at the making ready of the Prince, as well at night as in the morning, to see the assays taken as is aforesaid.

Item, that whatsoever new stuff, apparel, or raiment shall be brought of new to and for his grace's body, be it woollen, linen, silk, gold, or other kind whatsoever, or be new washed, before his grace shall wear any of the same, shall be purely brushed, made clean, aired at the fire, and perfumed thoroughly, so that the same way his grace may have no harm or displeasure, with assays taken from time to time as the case shall require, and that in the presence of the Chamberlain, Vice-chamberlain, or one of them.

Item, that no manner other persons or officers in the house shall have access to the said privy chamber, but only such as be appointed to the same; and that others which be appointed to bring in wood, make the fires, and other offices there, as the Pages of the chamber, incontinent as they shall have done their offices, shall depart and avoid out of the same, until the time they shall be called for the doing of their offices again; provided always that those pages shall not resort to any infect or corrupt places, and that also they shall be clean and whole persons without diseases.

Item, to avoid all infection and danger of pestilence and contagious diseases that might chance or happen in the Prince's household, by often resorting of the officers or servants of the same to London, to some infected and contagious places, his Majesty's said servants shall provide and put such order of as none of his grace's privy chamber, none of the officers that have any office about his grace's person or in his household shall resort to London, or to any other place, during the summer or contagious time; and if they shall for some necessary things have licence so to do, yet nevertheless after their return they shall abstain to resort to the Prince's grace presence, or to come near him for so many days, as by the said Chamberlain and Steward shall be thought convenient; and if by chance happen to any person to fall suddenly sick, that then without tract or delay of time to be removed out of the house.

Item, that forasmuch as the officers and other servants of his grace in the household, as well of kitchen, buttery, pantry, ewery, woodyard, cellar, larder, poultry, scalding house, saucer, yeomen, and grooms of the hall, have under them, as it is informed, sundry boys, pages, and servants, which without any respect go to and fro, and be not aware of the dangers of infection, and do often times resort unto suspect places; therefore the King's gracious pleasure is that, for the consequences which may follow of them, they shall be restrained from having any servant boy or page, and none to be admitted within the house.

Item, that such provision shall be taken as no infection may arise from the poor people, sore, and needy and sick resorting to his Grace's gate for alms; and for that purpose there shall be a place afar off appointed a good way from the gates, where the said poor people shall stay and tarry for the alms to be distributed there by the almoners, and after that distribution to depart accordingly; and if any beggar shall presume to draw near the gates, then they may be appointed to be gravely punished, to the example of others.

Item, that the said Steward and Chamberlain shall see good order to be kept in that household without and superfluous charges or waste, which is utterly to be avoided, so that the King's highness may in all points be put at the least charges that can be for that household; so that nevertheless the same may always be honourably kept as appertains; and that no manner of persons, of what degree so ever he or they be, shall have any more servants allowed within the Prince's house than to him shall be limited and appointed by an exchequer roll to the King's majesty's hand to be signed.

Item, that every officer within the Prince's household shall be sworn that they shall not serve the Prince's grace with any manner meat, drink, fruit, spice, or other thing whatsoever it be for his own person, but such as they shall serve every man in his own office, in his own person, suffering none other to meddle therewith, and before he or they shall so serve the Prince, shall, as well themselves as all others coming and having charge of the same, take and cause to be taken large assays from time to time, as the case shall require, and that the Chamberlain for the chamber, and the Steward for the household shall cause newly to be sworn all the Prince's servants at their first entry, of what condition, degree, or estate so ever they be of, for the due observation of their offices and duties as apply.

Appendix Two

The Sweating Sickness in Holinshed's *Chronicles*

The following extracts from Raphael Holinshed's *Chronicles*, originally published in 1577, are from J. Johnson's edition of 1808, issued as *Holinshed's Chronicles of England, Scotland*. They are taken from volume III, pp. 482, 536, 626, 735, 1031. The extracts have been lightly edited according to modern practice, for clarity.

[In 1485] a new kind of sickness invaded suddenly the people of this land, passing though the same from the one end to the other. It began about 21 September and continued until the latter end of October, being so sharp and deadly, that the like was never heard of to any man's remembrance before that time. For suddenly a deadly burning sweat so assailed their bodies and distempered their blood with a most ardent heat, that scarce one among a hundred that sickened did escape with his life: for all in a manner as soon as the sweat took them, or within a short time after, yielded the ghost. Beside the great number which deceased within the city of London, two mayors successively died within eight days and six aldermen.

At length, by the diligent observation of those that escaped (which marking what things had done them good, and helped their deliverance, used the like again), when they fell into the same disease the second or third time, as to divers it chanced, a remedy was found for that mortal malady, which was this. If a man in the daytime were taken with the sweat, then should he straight lie down with all his clothes and garments, and continue in his sweat for 24 hours, after so moderate a sort as might be. If in the night he chanced to be taken, then should he not rise out of his bed for the space of 24 hours, so casting the clothes that he might in no wise provoke the sweat, but lie so temperately, that the water might distil out softly of the own accord, and to abstain from all meat if he might so long suffer hunger, and to take no more drink either hot or cold, than would moderately quench and assuage his thirsty appetite. Thus with lukewarm drink, temperate heat, and measurable clothes many escaped: few which used this order (after it was found out) died of that sweat. Marry one point diligently above all other in this cure is to be observed, that he never did put his hand or feet out of the bed to refresh or cool himself, which to do is no less jeopardy than short and present death. Thus this disease coming in the first year of king Henry VII's reign, was judged (of some) to be a token and sign of a troublesome reign of the same king, as the proof partly afterwards showed itself.

[In 1506] the king began to be diseased of a certain infirmity... And because for the most part the harm that chances to the prince is [shared] with his subjects, the sweating sickness, which, as you have read in the first year of the reign of the king first afflicted the people of this realm, now assailed them again; howbeit by the remedy found at the beginning of it, nothing like the number died thereof now this second time, as did at the first time until the said remedy was invented.

[In 1518] in June the king had with him various ambassadors, for the entertainment of whom he prepared costly jousts...After this great triumph the king appointed his guests for his pastime this summer; but suddenly there came a plague of sickness, called the sweating sickness, that turned all his purpose.

This malady was so cruel, peremptory and deadly, that it killed some within three hours, some within two hours, some merry at dinner, and dead at supper. Many died in the king's court, the lord Clinton, the lord Grey of Wilton, and many knights, gentlemen, and officers. For this plague Michaelmas term was adjourned.

And because that this malady continued from July to the middle of December, the king kept himself ever with a small company, and held no solemn Christmas, willing to have no resort for fear of infection: but he much lamented the number of his people, for in some one town half the people died, and in some other town the third part, the sweat was so fervent and infectious. By the extremity whereof, and the multitudes with such suddenness and mortality dropping away, it should seem that they little remembered, or at least neglected, the preservative remedy used in the first great sweating sickness in king Henry VII's time, whereby many a man's life was saved, so now the like benefit, by application of the same wholesome means, might have benefited the patients.

[In 1528] in the end of May began in the city of London the disease called the sweating sickness, which afterwards infected all places of the realm, and slew many within five or six hours after they sickened. This sickness, for the manner of the taking of the patients, was an occasion of remembering that great sweat which raged in the reign of this king's father; and happily men caused the remedy then used to be revived. By reason of this sickness, the term was adjourned, and the circuit of the assizes also. There died divers in the court of this sickness, as Sir Francis Poynz, who had been ambassador in Spain, and divers others. The king for a space removed almost every day until he came to Tittenhanger, a place of the abbot of St Albans, and there he with the queen, and a small company about them, remained till the sickness was passed. In this great mortality died Sir William Compton knight, and William Carew, esquire; which were of the king's privy chamber.

[In 1551, in the reign of Edward VI]. At the end of the parliament, namely the 15 April the infectious sweating sickness began at Shrewsbury, which ended not in the north part of England until the end of September. In this space, what number died, it cannot be well accounted: but certain it is, that in London in a few days 960 gave up the ghost. It began in London the 9 July, and the 12 July it was most vehement: which was so terrible that people being in the best health, were suddenly taken and dead in 24 hours, and 12, or less, for lack of skill in guiding them in their sweat. And it is to be noted, that this mortality fell chiefly or rather upon men, and those also of the best age, as between 30 and 40 years. The speedy riddance of life procured by this sickness, did so terrify people of all sorts, that such as could make shift, with money or friendship, changed their soil, and leaving places of concourse, took themselves (for the time) to abodes, though not altogether solitary, yet less frequented: to conclude, manifold means were made for safety of life. The first week died in London 800 persons. Of this sweat died Henry and Charles sons of Charles Brandon, the elder first, and the younger after: so that they both died dukes of Suffolk.

The manner of this sweat was such, that if men did take any cold outwardly, it stroke the sweat in, and immediately killed them. If they were suffered to sleep, commonly they swooned in their sleep and departed, or else died immediately upon their waking. But the way to escape danger was close keeping moderately with some air and a little drink, and the same to be posset-ale, and so to keep them 30 hours, and then was the danger past; but beware of sudden cold. Before men had learned the manner of keeping, an infinite number perished. This disease at that time followed Englishmen and none other nation; for in Antwerp and other countries, our Englishmen being there among several other nations, only our Englishmen were sick thereof, and none other persons. The consideration of which thing made this nation much afraid thereof, who for the time began to repent and give alms, and to remember God from whom that plague might well seem to be sent among us. But as the disease in time ceased, so our devotion in short time decayed.

Notes

Chapter One
1. L&P, IV, 5825. John Gough, ed., *Chronicle of the Grey Friars of London*, Camden Soc., 53, 1852, p. 24.
2. Philip R. Liebson, 'The sweating sickness in Tudor England: a plague of the Renaissance', *Hektoen International Journal*, 5, 2013.
3. J.R. Lander, *The Wars of the Roses*, Stroud, Sutton, 2000, p. 209.
4. Philippe de Commynes, *Memoirs: The Reign of Louis XI 1461-83*, ed. Michael Jones, London, Penguin, 1972, p. 194.
5. Francis Bacon, *The History of the Reign of King Henry VII*, London, Hesperus, 2007, pp. 8-9. S.B. Chrimes, *Henry VII*, London and New Haven, Yale UP, 1999, p. 52.
6. John L. Flood, "Safer on the battlefield than in the city': England, the "sweating sickness" and the continent', *Renaissance Studies*, 17, 2003, p. 164.
7. John Noorthouck, *A New History of London Including Westminster and Southwark*, London, 1773, bk 1, ch. 7.
8. Shakespeare, *Measure for Measure*, act 1 sc 2, ed. Jonathan Bate and Eric Rasmussen, London, Macmillan, 2010, p. 27.
9. Paul Heyman, Leopold Simons and Christel Cochez, 'Were the English Sweating Sickness and the Picardy Sweat Caused by Hantaviruses?', *Viruses*, 6, 2014, p. 153. Arno Karlen, *Plague's Progress: A Social History of Man and Disease*, London, Gollancz, 1995, p. 81.
10. Thomas Forestier, *Tractatus contra pestilentiam thenasmonem et dissinteriam*, Rouen, 1490. BL, Add MSS 27,582, ff. 70-7. Lori Jones, Exploring Concepts of Contagion and the Authority of Medical Treatises in 14th-16th century England, MA thesis, University of Ottawa, 2012, pp. 48, 71, 80, 82. Carole Rawcliffe, 'Health and Safety at Work', in Christopher Harper-Bill, ed., *Medieval East Anglia*, Woodbridge, Boydell, 2005, p. 139. Carole Rawcliffe, *Urban Bodies; Communal Health in Late Medieval English Towns and Cities*, Woodbridge, Boydell, 2013, pp. 100, 188.
11. John Caius, *A boke, or counseill against the disease commonly called the sweate or sweating sicknesse*, London, 1552, p. 8.
12. *CSPVen, V, 1534-1554*, item 534.

13. *Correspondence of Erasmus*, 5, p. 68.
14. L&P, IV, 4710. W.K. Jordan, ed., *The Chronicle and Political Papers of King Edward VI*, London, George Allen & Unwin, 1966, p. 71.
15. Hall, *Chronicle*, II, p. 137. Polydore Vergil, *The Anglica Historia 1485-1537*, in Roger Lockyer, *Henry VII*, London, Longman, 1968, p. 110. L&P, IV, 4710.
16. *Westminster Review*, 1871, p. 45.
17. Caius, *A boke or counseill*, p. 17.
18. Mrs Henry Cust, *Gentlemen Errant, being the journeys of four noblemen in Europe during the fifteenth and sixteenth centuries*, London, John Murray, 1909, p. 337. L&P, IV, 4510.
19. L&P, IV, 4710.
20. Roger Lockyer, *Henry VII*, London, Longman, 1968, p. 110. L&P, II, App. to Preface; IV, 4440. John Lyly, *Galatea*, ed. George K. Hunter, Manchester, Manchester UP, 2000, p. 36.
21. Bacon, *King Henry VII*, pp. 9-10.
22. Caius, *A boke or counseill*, p. 30.
23. L&P, IV, 4710.
24. L&P, II, App. to Preface.
25. L&P, II, App. to Preface.
26. Caius, *A boke or counseill*, p. 19.
27. L&P, IV, 4510.
28. Bacon, *King Henry VII*, p. 10.

Chapter Two
1. Dorothy H. Crawford, *Deadly Companions: How Microbes Shaped Our History*, Oxford, OUP, 2007, p. 125.
2. Crawford, *Deadly Companions*, p. 66. Reginald R. Sharpe, ed., *Calendar of Letter-Books...of the City of London, L*, Corporation of London, 1912, pp. 102-3. Philip E. Jones, ed., *Calendar of Plea and Memoranda Rolls, 1458-1482*, Cambridge, CUP, 1961, p. 102.
3. *Correspondence of Erasmus*, 6, pp. 39, 41.
4. Francis Bacon, *The History of the Reign of King Henry VII*, London, Hesperus, 2007, p. 9.
5. Jon Arrizabalaga, John Henderson and Roger French, *The Great Pox: The French Disease in Renaissance Europe*, New Haven & London, Yale UP, 1997, p. 88.
6. Marie Collins, ed., *Caxton, The Description of Britain*, London, Weidenfeld & Nicolson, 1988, pp. 117-18.
7. Thomas More, *Utopia*, trans Paul Turner, London, Penguin, 2009, p. 17.
8. Hall *Chronicle*, I, p. 320; II p. 38.
9. *Correspondence of Erasmus*, 2, p. 129.

Chapter Three

1. Thomas More, *Utopia*, trans Paul Turner, London, Penguin, 2009, p. 63.
2. John Caius, *A boke or counseill against the disease commonly called the sweate or sweatyng sicknesse*, 1552, p. xx.
3. Roger Lockyer, ed., *Thomas Wolsey late Cardinal his Life and Death written by George Cavendish*, London, Folio Soc., 1963, p. 51.
4. *Westminster Review*, 1871, p. 45.
5. C.H. Williams, *English Historical Documents 1485-1558*, London, Eyre & Spottiswood, 1967, p. 189. Lori Jones, Exploring Concepts of Contagion and the Authority of Medical Treatises in 14th-16th century England, MA thesis, University of Ottawa, 2012, p. 46.
6. *Westminster Review*, 1871, p. 45.
7. E.F. Rogers, *St Thomas More: Selected Letters*, London & New Haven, Yale UP, 1961, pp. 4-5.
8. H. Edmund Poole, ed., *The Wisdom of Andrew Boorde*, Leicester, Edgar Backus, 1936, pp. 21, 51-2. *Westminster Review*, 1871, p. 45. Thompson, *Collected Works of Erasmus, Colloquies*, vol. 1, p. 721 n. 8.
9. C.V. Malfatti, ed., *Two Italian Accounts of Tudor England. A Journey to London in 1497*, Barcelona, C.V. Malfatti, 1953.
10. Dominic Mancini, *The Usurpation of Richard the Third*, ed. C.A.J. Armstrong, Gloucester, Sutton, 1989, p. 103.
11. L&P, III, 1519-23, 3657. CSPVen, 5, 1534-1554, 934.
12. Lucy Toulmin Smith, ed., *The Itinerary of John Leland in or about the Years 1535-1543*, London, George Bell & Son, 1907–10, I, pp. 7, 74, III, pp. 228, 254, 270.
13. W.G. Hoskins, 'The Elizabethan Merchants of Exeter', in Peter Clark, ed., *The Early Modern Town*, London, Longman, 1976, p. 159.
14. Alan D. Dyer, *The City of Worcester in the Sixteenth Century*, Leicester, Leicester UP, 1973, p. 206. Mary Dormer Harris, ed., *The Coventry Leet Book: or Mayor's Register 1420-1555*, Early English Text Soc., 1907-13, p. 652.
15. J.G. Nichols, ed., *Chronicle of the Grey Friars of London*, Camden Soc., 53, 1852, pp. 26-7.
16. Rawdon Brown, *Four Years at the Court of Henry VIII*, London, Smith, Elder, 1854, I, p. 110.
17. Lockyer, ed., *Thomas Wolsey*, p. 53.
18. G.W. Groos, ed., *The Diary of Baron Waldstein. A Traveller in Elizabethan England*, London, Thames & Hudson, 1981, p. 43.
19. Polydore Vergil, *The Anglica Historia 1485-1537*, in Roger Lockyer, *Henry VII*, London, Longman, 1968, p. 110.
20. Simon Thurley, *The Royal Palaces of Tudor England*, London & New Haven, Yale UP, 1993, pp. 67-70.
21. Charles Creighton, *A History of Epidemics in Britain (Volume I of II) from A.D. 664 to the Extinction of Plague*, Cambridge, CUP, 1891, pp. 242-3.

22. L&P, IV, item 2343.
23. George Clark, *A History of the Royal College of Physicians of London*, I, Oxford, Clarendon Press, 1964, pp. 6, 17-18.
24. Clark, *Royal College*, pp. 54-5.
25. Desiderius Erasmus, *Praise of Folly*, trans Betty Radice, London, Penguin, 1993, p. 52.
26. *Correspondence of Erasmus*, 4, p. 405.
27. Caius, *A boke or counseill*, p. 26.
28. Thurley, *Royal Palaces*, pp. 69-70.
29. Brown *Four Years*, I, p. 262.
30. Tim Coates, ed., *Letters of Henry VIII, 1526-29*, London, HMSO, 2001, p. 193.
31. *Correspondence of Erasmus*, 5, pp. 319, 353.
32. Daniel Defoe, *A Journal of the Plague Year*, ed. Cynthia Wall, London, Penguin, 2003, pp. 26-8.

Chapter Four
1. R.S. Gottfried, 'Population, Plague, and the Sweating Sickness: Demographic Movements in Late Fifteenth-Century England', *Journal of British Studies*, 17, 1977, pp. 20-1. John L. Flood, "Safer on the battlefield than in the city': England, the "sweating sickness", and the continent', *Renaissance Studies*, 17, 2003, pp. 148, 162. Henry Ellis, ed., *The Chronicle of John Hardyng*, London, 1812, p. 550.
2. Simon Thurley, *Houses of Power: The Places That Shaped the Tudor World*, London, Bantam Press, 2017, p. 12.
3. Charles Creighton, *A History of Epidemics in Britain*, Cambridge, CUP, 1891, pp. 239-43.
4. Wills: 1-2 Richard III (1483-5), in R.R. Sharpe, ed., *Calendar of Wills Proved and Enrolled in the Court of Husting, London: Part 2, 1358-1688*, London, 1890, pp. 585-8, n.5.
5. TNA, PROB 11/7/236. John Stow, *The Survey of London*, ed. H.B. Wheatley, Dent, London, 1987, p. 190.
6. Thomas Allen, *The History and Antiquities of London, Westminster, Southwark, and ...*, Volume 3, London, Cowie & Strange, 1828, p. 148. TNA, PROB 11/7/230.
7. H.T. Riley, *Ingulph's Chronicle of the Abbey of Croyland*, London, Henry G. Bohn, 1854, p. 495. James Gairdner, *The Paston Letters, A.D. 1422-1509*, VI, London, Chatto & Windus, 1904, p. 86.
8. Gottfried, 'Population, Plague and the Sweating Sickness', pp. 18, 21, 22, 25, 35.
9. J.F.D. Shrewsbury, *A History of Bubonic Plague in the British Isles*, Cambridge, CUP, 1970, p. 159.
10. Lucy Toulmin Smith, ed., *The Itinerary of John Leland in or about the Years 1535-1543*, London, George Bell & Son, 1907–10, II, p. 77.

11. Caroline Skeel, *The Council in the Marches of Wales: A Study in Local Government during the Sixteenth and Seventeenth centuries*, London, H. Rees, 1904, p. 30.
12. Toulmin Smith, ed., *Itinerary of John Leland*, II, p. 78.
13. *Cal. State Papers, Spain, Volume 1, 1485-1509*, items 319, 321, 322, 324.
14. Francis Bacon, *The History of the Reign of King Henry VII*, London, Hesperus, 2007, p. 142.
15. E.W. Ives, 'Henry VIII (1491–1547)', *ODNB*.
16. John Guy, *The Children of Henry VIII*, Oxford, OUP, 2013, Prologue. Thomas Penn, *Winter King: The Dawn of Tudor England*, London, Penguin, 2011, p. 70.
17. Sean Cunningham, *Prince Arthur: The Tudor King Who Never Was*, Stroud, Amberley, 2016, pp. 171-4.
18. John Stow, *Annales, or a Generall Chronicle of England*, London, 1631, p. 485.
19. *An Essay Towards A Topographical History of the County of Norfolk: Volume 3, the History of the City and County of Norwich, Part I.* London, W. Miller, 1806, Chap XXII.
20. J.S. Barrow, J.D. Herson, A.H. Lawes, P.J. Riden and M.V.J. Seaborne, 'Economic infrastructure and institutions: Population', in A.T. Thacker and C.P. Lewis, eds, *A History of the County of Chester, Volume 5 Part 2, the City of Chester: Culture, Buildings, Institutions*, London, 2005, pp. 71-3.
21. VCH, *Norfolk*, II, London, 1906, pp. 370-2.
22. Creighton, *History of Epidemics in Britain*, pp. 244-5. Penn, *Winter King*, p. 324.
23. Geoffrey Parker, *Emperor: A New Life of Charles V*, London & New Haven, Yale UP, 2019, p. 21.
24. *The Will of King Henry VII*, London, T. Payne, 1775, pp. 15-19.

Chapter Five
1. Hall, *Chronicle*, I, p. 14.
2. *Correspondence of Erasmus*, II, pp. 147-8.
3. *Correspondence of Erasmus*, II, pp. 182, 199.
4. *Correspondence of Erasmus*, II, pp. 169, 176, 182, 189.
5. *Correspondence of Erasmus*, II, pp. 252, 259, 260. L&P. I, 2412. *CSPVen*, II, items 333, 340, 353, 360.
6. *Correspondence of Erasmus*, II, p. 277. F.A. Inderwick, ed., *A Calendar of the Inner Temple Records, I, 1505-1603*, London, 1896, p. 28.
7. L&P, I, item 2929.
8. J.G. Nichols, ed., *Chronicle of the Grey Friars of London*, Camden Soc., 53, 1852, p. 29.
9. L&P, II, items 1815, 1832.
10. Rawdon Brown, *Four Years at the Court of Henry VIII*, London, Smith, Elder, 1854, II, pp. 69-75.

11. Hall, *Chronicle*, I, pp. 157-63. Nichols, ed., *Chronicle of the Grey Friars*, p. 30.
12. Hall, *Chronicle*, I, p. 165. Brown, *Four Years*, II, pp. 113-15.
13. *Correspondence of Erasmus*, 5, pp. 68-9, 88.
14. *Four Years*, II, pp. 126-9. *CSPVen*, II, items 945, 950, 958, 959.
15. Inderwick, ed., *Inner Temple Records, I*, p. 41.
16. J.R. Hale, ed., *The Travel Journal of Antonio de Beatis*, London, Hakluyt Soc., 1979, pp. 9-11, 104. L&P, II, item 3572.
17. J.B. Trapp, 'Ammonius, Andreas [Andrea della Rena], (bap. 1476, d. 1517)', *ODNB*. *Correspondence of Erasmus*, 5, pp. 68-9, 88-9.
18. Brown, *Four Years*, II, pp. 130, 135, 139-40, 142.
19. Hall, *Chronicle*, I, p. 165.
20. Euan C. Roger, "To Be Shut Up': New Evidence for the Development of Quarantine Regulations in Early-Tudor England', *Social History of Medicine*, April 2019, pp. 1-20.
21. R.W. Heinze, *Proclamations of the Tudor Kings*, Cambridge, CUP, 1976, p. 104.
22. L&P, II, item 4125.
23. F.P. Wilson, *The Plague in Shakespeare's London*, Oxford, OUP, 1927, p. 62.
24. L&P, II, item 4320. *Correspondence of Erasmus*, V, pp. 306, 335.
25. Chris Tremlett, *Catherine of Aragon: Henry's Spanish Queen*, London, Faber & Faber, 2010, p. 225.
26. Brown, *Four Years*, II, pp. 201-3.

Chapter Six
1. David Loades, *Mary Tudor*, Stroud, Amberley, 2012, pp. 24-5.
2. Hall, *Chronicle*, II, p. 56.
3. John Caius, *A boke or counseill against the disease commonly called the sweate or sweatyng sicknesse*, 1552, p. 11.
4. Hall, *Chronicle*, II, p. 137. John Stow, *Annales, or a general Chronicle of England*, 1631, p. 923.
5. Tim Coates, ed., *Letters of Henry VIII, 1526-29*, London, HMSO, 2001, pp. 56-8.
6. L&P, IV, item 4422.
7. L&P, IV, items 4408, 4440, 4463, 4476, 4486, 4489. Hall, *Chronicle*, II, p. 137. Francis C. Webb, *The Sweating Sickness in England*, London, 1857, pp. 10-11. David Gordon and Peter Gordon, *Musical Visitors to Britain*, London, Routledge, 2007, pp. 17-18.
8. L&P, IV, items 4417, 4453, 4542, 4604.
9. L&P, IV, item 4656.
10. Tracy Borman, *Henry VIII and the men who made him*, London, Hodder & Stoughton, 2018, pp. 74-5, 118, 136, 150-1, 154-5. G.W. Bernard,

'Compton, Sir William (1482?–1528)'; Michael Riordan, 'Carey, William (c. 1496–1528)', *ODNB*.
11. L&P, IV, item 4493, 4690. Susan Brigden, *London and the Reformation*, London, Faber & Faber, 2014, p. 139.
12. Webb, *Sweating Sickness*, pp. 10-11. L&P, IV, items 4510, 4542, 4891, 5191.
13. L&P, IV, 4633.
14. L&P, IV, app. 180.
15. *CSPVen*, IV, item 364.
16. *State Papers: Volume I, King Henry the Eighth, Parts 1. and 2.*, London, 1830, pp. 385-6. Reginald H. Adams, *The Parish Clerks of London*, London and Chichester, Phillimore, 1971, p. 48.
17. Adams, *Parish Clerks*, p. 49.
18. L&P, IV, item 4510.
19. John Christiansen, 'The English Sweat in Lübeck and North Germany, 1529', *Medical History*, 53, 2009, pp. 416, 419.
20. Johannes Janssen, *History of the German People at the Close of the Middle Ages*, XIV, London, Kegan Paul, 1909, p. 61.
21. David Daniell, *William Tyndale: A Biography*, London & New Haven, Yale UP, 1994, p. 198.
22. Jennifer Jenkins, *Provincial Modernity: Local Culture and Liberal Politics in Fin-de-Siècle Hamburg*, Ithaca & London, Cornell UP, 2003, p. 23.
23. John Christiansen, 'The English Sweat in Lübeck and North Germany, 1529', *Medical History*, 53, 2009, pp. 417-18, 422-3. Flood, 'Safer on the battlefield', p. 175. Mrs Henry Cust, *Gentlemen Errant, being the journeys of four noblemen in Europe during the fifteenth and sixteenth centuries*, London, John Murray, 1909, pp. 337-8.
24. Creighton, *History of Epidemics*, I, p. 265. Flood, 'Safer on the battlefield', pp. 160-1.
25. Christiansen, 'English Sweat', p. 417.
26. Flood, 'Safer on the battlefield', pp. 159-60.
27. Claudia Resch, "The English Sweating Sickness' of 1529 in Augsburg: A Challenge to Body and Soul and the Printer', 2009, English abstract. Creighton, *History of Epidemics*, I, p. 258.
28. Paul Arblaster, Gergely Juhász and Guido Latré, eds, *Tyndale's Testament*, Turnhout, Brepols, 2002, pp. 140-1.
29. Flood, 'Safer on the battlefield', p. 158.
30. Flood, 'Safer on the battlefield, pp. 170-1.
31. Creighton, *History of Epidemics*, I, pp. 156-7. Flood, 'Safer on the battlefield', p. 161.
32. Flood, 'Safer on the battlefield', pp. 156-7.

Chapter Seven

1. Desiderius Erasmus, *Praise of Folly*, trans Betty Radice, London, Penguin, 1993, p. 77.
2. H. Edmund Poole, *The Wisdome of Andrew Boorde*, Leicester, Falconer Scott, 1936, p. 51.
3. Tracy Borman, *Henry VIII and the men who made him*, London, Hodder & Stoughton, 2018, pp. 168, 229.
4. L&P, V, 1533, items 948, 975, 1000, 1047, 1049, 1063.
5. L&P, 12, item 298.
6. Simon Lambe, 'Life in the Time of Plague', *History Today*, 70/7, July 2020, pp. 14-15. W.K. Jordan, *The Chronicle and Political Papers of King Edward VI*, London, Allen & Unwin, 1966, p. 3.
7. Simon Thurley, *The Royal Palaces of Tudor England*, London & New Haven, Yale UP, 1993. L&P, XIV pt 1, item 517.
8. John Gough Nicols, ed., *Literary Remains of King Edward the Sixth*, I, London, Roxburghe Club, 1857, pp. xxvii-xxx. Borman, *Henry VIII*, p. 319.
9. Nichols, ed., *Literary Remains*, I, p. xxix.
10. Borman, *Henry VIII*, p. 369. L&P, XVI, item 1297.
11. Paul L. Hughes and James F. Larkin, eds., *Tudor Royal Proclamations Volume I The Early Tudors (1485-1553)*, London & New Haven, Yale UP, 1964, pp. 319-20, 339.
12. Thomas Vicary, *The Anatomie of the Bodie of Man*, ed. Frederick J. Furnivall and Percy Furnivall, Early English Text Soc., extra series, 53, 1888, pp. 160-1.
13. Vicary, *Anatomie*, p. 117.
14. *CSPVen*, vol. 15, 1534-54, p. 542. John Stow and Edmond Howes, *The annales, or generall chronicle of England*, 1615, p. 605. Jordan, ed., *Chronicle and Political Papers*, p. 71. John Caius, *A boke or counseill against the disease commonly called the sweate or sweatyng sicknesse*, London, 1552, pp. 11-12. J.G. Nichols, ed., *The Diary of Henry Machyn Citizen and Merchant-Taylor of London (1550-1563)*, Camden Soc., 1848, pp. 7-8, 318-19. J.G. Nichols, ed., *Chronicle of the Grey Friars of London*, Camden Soc., vol.53, 1852, p. 70.
15. Francis C. Webb, 'The Sweating Sickness in England', *The Sanitary Review and Journal of Public Health*, III, 1857, p. 122. J.V. Kitto, ed., *St Martin-in-The-Fields: the Accounts of the Churchwardens, 1525-1603*, London, 1901, pp. 134-40. J. Charles Cox, *The Parish registers of England*, London, Methuen, 1910, pp. 143-4.
16. Stow, *Annales*, p. 605. Natalie Mears and Alec Ryrie, eds, *Worship and the Parish Church in Early Modern Britain*, London, Routledge, 2016, p. 36.
17. Alan D. Dyer, *The City of Worcester in the sixteenth century*, Leicester, Leicester UP, 1973, p. 44. A.T. Thacker and C.P. Lewis, eds, *VCH Cheshire: Vol. 5 pt 2, the City of Chester*, London, 2005, pp. 71-3.

18. Alan Dyer, 'The English Sweating Sickness of 1551: an Epidemic Anatomized', *Medical History*, 41, 1997, pp. 365-6. E.A. Wrigley and R.S. Schofield, *The Population History of England 1541-1871, A Reconstruction*, Cambridge, CUP, 1981, p. 337.
19. Webb, 'Sweating Sickness', p. 121.
20. Paul Slack, 'The Local Incidence of Epidemic Disease: the Case of Bristol 1540-1650', *The Plague Reconsidered*, Local Population Studies Supplement, 1977, pp. 49-51.
21. Webb, 'Sweating Sickness', p. 122.
22. Nicols, ed., *Literary Remains*, II, p. 330, n. 1.
23. J.F.D. Shrewsbury, *A History of Bubonic Plague in the British Isles*, Cambridge, CUP, 1970, p. 185. John Jones, *A Dyall for all Agues*, London, 1566, unpaged.
24. S.J. Gunn, 'Brandon, Charles, first duke of Suffolk (c. 1484–1545)', *ODNB*.
25. Dyer, 'English Sweating Sickness of 1551', pp. 367-74. Caius, *A boke or counseill against the Sweat*, p. 9.
26. W.D. Robson-Scott, *German Travellers in England 1400-1800*, Oxford, Blackwell, 1953, pp. 27-30.
27. Nicols, ed., *Literary Remains*, p. 87.
28. Alan D. Dyer, 'The Influence of Bubonic Plague in England 1500-1667', *Medical History*, 22, 1978, p. 324.
29. TNA, SP10/13/30 f. 62.
30. Diarmaid MacCulloch, *Thomas Cranmer: A Life*, London & New Haven, Yale UP, 2016 edn, pp. 483, 487. Dirk W. Rodgers, 'À Lasco [Laski], John (1499–1560)', *ODNB*.
31. Charles F. Mullett, *The Bubonic Plague and England: An Essay in the History of Preventive Medicine*, Lexington, University of Kentucky Press, 1956, p. 57. Charles Nevinson, *Later Writings of Bishop Hooper*, Parker Soc., 1852, pp. 57, 165-7.
32. Webb, 'Sweating Sickness', p. 123.
33. *CSPVen*, vol.5, 1534-1554, item 934.
34. Jared Bernard, 'The Dreaded Sweat: the Other Medieval Epidemic', *History Today*, May 2014.
35. Jones, *Dyall for all Agues*, unpaged.

Chapter Eight
1. Mary Hill Cole, *The Portable Queen: Elizabeth I and the Politics of Ceremony*, Amherst, University of Massachusetts Press, 1999, pp. 20-1.
2. Carole Levine, 'Faunt, Nicholas (1553/4–1608)', *ODNB*. Lisa Jardine and Alan Stewart, *Hostage to Fortune: The Troubled Life of Francis Bacon, 1561-1626*, London, Gollancz, 1998, pp. 84-7, 89.
3. Thomas Birch, *Memoirs of the Reign of Queen Elizabeth I*, London, 1754, p. 31.

4. Desmond MacCarthy, ed., *The Essayes of Michael Lord of Montaigne translated into English by John Florio*, I, London & Toronto, Dent, 1928, p. 81.
5. *Analytical Index to...The Remembrancia...of the City of London, A.D. 1579-1664*, London, E.J. Francis, 1878, p. 337.
6. *Analytical Index to...The Remembrancia*, pp. 336-7.
7. LMA, Common Council Journal XXI f. 283v.
8. Patricia Basing and Dennis E. Rhodes, 'English plague regulations and Italian models: printed and manuscript items in the Yelverton collection', *British Library Journal*, 23, 1997, pp. 60-7.
9. LMA, Common Council Journal XXI, ff. 285r-6v. W.P. Barrett, *Present Remedies against the Plague*, London, Shakespeare Association Facsimiles No. 7, 1933, pp. viii-xiii.
10. LMA, Common Council Journal XXI, f. 199v.
11. Cyndia Susan Clegg, 'Holinshed [Hollingshead], Raphael, (c. 1525–1580?)', *ODNB*.
12. J. Johnson, ed., *Holinshed's Chronicles of England, Scotland*, III, London, 1808, pp. 482, 536, 626, 735, 1031.
13. *APC, 40, 1625-1626*, p. 13.
14. *CSPD, 1635-1636*, p. 523; *1636-1637*, pp. 126, 130.
15. Wellcome Collection, Tom Ruby being tricked by six friends into thinking he is suffering from the 'sweating sickness'. Coloured line engraving, 1799.
16. Francis C. Webb, 'The Sweating Sickness in England', *Sanitary Review Journal of Public Health*, 3, 1857, p. 108.
17. Charles Creighton, *A History of Epidemics in Britain (Volume I of II) from A.D. 664 to the Extinction of Plague*, Cambridge, CUP 1891, p. 266.
18. John Caius, *A boke or counseill against the disease commonly called the sweate or sweatyng sicknesse*, 1552, pp. 11-12.
19. J.F.D. Shrewsbury, *A History of Bubonic Plague in the British Isles*, Cambridge, CUP, 1970, pp. 180, 184-5. Alan Dyer, 'The English Sweating Sickness of 1551: an Epidemic Anatomized', *Medical History*, 41, 1997, pp. 362-84.
20. George Clark, *A History of the Royal College of Physicians of London*, I, Oxford, Clarendon Press, 1964, p. 108. Robert S. Gottfried, *Epidemic Disease in Fifteenth Century England*, Leicester, Leicester UP, 1978, p. 62. Mrs Henry Cust, *Gentlemen Errant, being the journeys of four noblemen in Europe during the fifteenth and sixteenth centuries*, London, John Murray, 1909, pp. 337-8.
21. Susan Scott and Christopher J. Duncan, *Biology of Plagues: Evidence from Historical Populations*, Cambridge, CUP, 2001, pp. 149-52. Michael B.A. Oldstone, *Viruses, Plagues and History*, 2nd edn., Oxford, OUP, 2020, p. 287. J.A.H. Wylie and L.H. Collier, 'The English Sweating Sickness (sudor anglicus): a reappraisal', *Journal of the History of Medicine*, 36, 1981, pp. 425-45. Paul Heyman, Leopold Simons and Christel Cochez,

'Were the English Sweating Sickness and the Picardy Sweat Caused by Hantavirus?', *Viruses*, 6, 2014, pp. 151-71. Paul Heyman, Christel Cochez and Mirsada Hukić, 'The English Sweating Sickness: Out of Sight, Out of Mind?', *Acta Medica Academica*, 47, 2018, pp. 102-116.
22. Heyman et al., 'English Sweating Sickness', pp. 151-61. Dyer, 'English Sweating Sickness of 1551', pp. 379, 383.
23. W.K. Jordan, ed., *The Chronicle and Political Papers of King Edward VI*, London, George Allen & Unwin, 1966, p. 71.

Bibliography

Adams, Reginald H., *The Parish Clerks of London*, London and Chichester, Phillimore, 1971

Allen, Thomas, *The History and Antiquities of London, Westminster, Southwark, and ...*, Volume 3, London, Cowie & Strange, 1828

Arrizabalaga, Jon, Henderson, John, and French, Roger, *The Great Pox: The French Disease in Renaissance Europe*, New Haven & London, Yale UP, 1997

Bacon, Francis, *The History of the Reign of King Henry VII*, London, Hesperus, 2007

Barrett, W.P., *Present Remedies against the Plague*, London, Shakespeare Association Facsimiles No. 7, 1933

Basing, Patricia, and Rhodes, Dennis E., 'English plague regulations and Italian models: printed and manuscript items in the Yelverton collection', *British Library Journal*, 23, 1997

Bernard, G.W., 'Compton, Sir William (1482?–1528)', *ODNB*

Bernard, Jared, 'The Dreaded Sweat: the Other Medieval Epidemic', *History Today*, May 2014

Birch, Thomas, *Memoirs of the Reign of Queen Elizabeth I*, London, 1754

Borman, Tracy, *Henry VIII and the men who made him*, London, Hodder & Stoughton, 2018

Brigden, Susan, *London and the Reformation*, London, Faber & Faber, 2014

Brown, Rawdon, *Four Years at the Court of Henry VIII*, London, Smith, Elder, 1854

Byrne, Muriel St.Clare, *The Lisle Letters, An Abridgement*, London, Secker & Warburg, 1983

Caius, John, *A boke or counseill against the disease commonly called the sweate or sweatyng sicknesse*, 1552

Chrimes, S.B., *Henry VII*, London and New Haven, Yale UP, 1999

Christiansen, John, 'The English Sweat in Lübeck and North Germany, 1529', *Medical History*, 53, 2009

Clark, George, *A History of the Royal College of Physicians of London*, I, Oxford, Clarendon Press, 1964

Clark, Peter, ed., *The Early Modern Town*, London, Longman, 1976

Clegg, Cyndia Susan, 'Holinshed [Hollingshead], Raphael, (c. 1525–1580?)', *ODNB*

Coates, Tim, ed., *Letters of Henry VIII, 1526-29*, London, HMSO, 2001
Cole, Mary Hill, *The Portable Queen: Elizabeth I and the Politics of Ceremony*, Amherst, University of Massachusetts Press, 1999
Collins, Marie, ed., *Caxton, The Description of Britain*, London, Weidenfeld & Nicolson, 1988
Commynes, Philippe de, *Memoirs: The Reign of Louis XI 1461-83*, ed. Michael Jones, London, Penguin, 1972
Cox, J. Charles, *The Parish registers of England*, London, Methuen, 1910
Crawford, Dorothy H., *Deadly Companions: How Microbes Shaped Our History*, Oxford, OUP, 2007
Creighton, Charles, *A History of Epidemics in Britain (Volume I of II) from A.D. 664 to the Extinction of Plague*, Cambridge, CUP, 1891
Cunningham, Sean, *Prince Arthur: The Tudor King Who Never Was*, Stroud, Amberley, 2016
Cust, Mrs Henry, *Gentlemen Errant, being the journeys of four noblemen in Europe during the fifteenth and sixteenth centuries*, London, John Murray, 1909
Daniell, David, *William Tyndale: A Biography*, London & New Haven, Yale UP, 1994
de Beer, Sir Gavin, *Early Travellers in the Alps*, London, Sidgwick & Jackson, 1966
Defoe, Daniel, *A Journal of the Plague Year*, ed. Cynthia Wall, London, Penguin, 2003
Dyer, Alan D., *The City of Worcester in the sixteenth century*, Leicester, Leicester UP, 1973
Dyer, Alan D., 'The Influence of Bubonic Plague in England 1500-1667', *Medical History*, 22, 1978
Dyer, Alan, 'The English Sweating Sickness of 1551: an Epidemic Anatomized', *Medical History*, 41, 1997
Ellis, Henry, ed., *The Chronicle of John Hardyng*, London, 1812
Erasmus, Desiderius, *Praise of Folly*, trans Betty Radice, London, Penguin, 1993
Flood, John L., "Safer on the battlefield than in the city': England, the "sweating sickness" and the continent', *Renaissance Studies*, 17, 2003
Gairdner, James, *The Paston Letters, A.D. 1422-1509*, VI, London, Chatto & Windus, 1904
Gordon, David and Gordon, Peter, *Musical Visitors to Britain*, London, Routledge, 2007
Gottfried, Robert S., *Epidemic Disease in Fifteenth Century England*, Leicester, Leicester UP, 1978
Gottfried, R.S., 'Population, Plague, and the Sweating Sickness: Demographic Movements in Late Fifteenth-Century England', *Journal of British Studies*, 17, 1977
Gough, John, ed., *Chronicle of the Grey Friars of London*, Camden Soc., 53, 1852

Groos, G.W., ed., *The Diary of Baron Waldstein. A Traveller in Elizabethan England*, London, Thames & Hudson, 1981

Gunn, S.J., 'Brandon, Charles, first duke of Suffolk (c. 1484–1545)', *ODNB*

Guy, John, *The Children of Henry VIII*, Oxford, OUP, 2013

Hale, J.R., ed., *The Travel Journal of Antonio de Beatis*, London, Hakluyt Soc., 1979

Hall, Edward, *[Chronicle].The Lives of the Kings. By Edward Hall* ed. C. Whibley, 2 vols. London, T.C. and E.C. Jack, 1904

Harper-Bill, Christopher, ed., *Medieval East Anglia*, Woodbridge, Boydell, 2005

Harris, Mary Dormer, ed., *The Coventry Leet Book: or Mayor's Register 1420-1555*, Early English Text Soc., 1907-13

Heinze, R.W., *Proclamations of the Tudor Kings*, Cambridge, CUP, 1976

Henry VII: *The Will of King Henry VII*, London, T. Payne, 1775

Heyman, Paul, Cochez, Christel, and Hukić, Mirsada, 'The English Sweating Sickness: Out of Sight, Out of Mind?', *Acta Medica Academica*, 47, 2018

Heyman, Paul, Simons, Leopold, and Cochez, Christel, 'Were the English Sweating Sickness and the Picardy Sweat Caused by Hantaviruses?', *Viruses*, 6, 2014

Hughes, Paul L., and Larkin, James F., eds., *Tudor Royal Proclamations Volume I The Early Tudors (1485-1553)*, London & New Haven, Yale UP, 1964

Inderwick, F.A., ed., *A Calendar of the Inner Temple Records, I, 1505-1603*, London, 1896

Janssen, Johannes, *History of the German People at the Close of the Middle Ages*, XIV, London, Kegan Paul, 1909

Jardine, Lisa, and Stewart, Alan, *Hostage to Fortune: The Troubled Life of Francis Bacon, 1561-1626*, London, Gollancz, 1998

Jenkins, Jennifer, *Provincial Modernity: Local Culture and Liberal Politics in Fin-de-Siècle Hamburg*, Ithaca & London, Cornell UP, 2003

Johnson, J., ed., *Holinshed's Chronicles of England, Scotland*, London, 1808

Jones, John, *A Dyall for all Agues*, London, 1566

Jones, Lori, Exploring Concepts of Contagion and the Authority of Medical Treatises in 14th-16th century England, MA thesis, University of Ottawa, 2012

Jones, Philip E., ed., *Calendar of Plea and Memoranda Rolls, 1458-1482*, Cambridge, CUP, 1961

Jordan, W.K., ed., *The Chronicle and Political Papers of King Edward VI*, London, George Allen & Unwin, 1966

Karlen, Arno, *Plague's Progress: A Social History of Man and Disease*, London, Gollancz, 1995

Kitto, J.V., ed., *St Martin-in-The-Fields: the Accounts of the Churchwardens, 1525-1603*, London, 1901

Lambe, Simon, 'Life in the Time of Plague', *History Today*, 70/7, July 2020

Lander, J.R., *The Wars of the Roses*, Stroud, Sutton, 2000
Levine, Carole, 'Faunt, Nicholas (1553/4–1608)', *ODNB*
Liebson, Philip R., 'The sweating sickness in Tudor England: a plague of the Renaissance', *Hektoen International Journal*, 5, 2013
Loades, David, *Mary Tudor*, Stroud, Amberley, 2012
Lockyer, Roger, ed., *Thomas Wolsey late Cardinal his Life and Death written by George Cavendish*, London, Folio Soc., 1963
Lockyer, Roger, *Henry VII*, London, Longman, 1968
Lyly, John, *Galatea*, ed. George K. Hunter, Manchester, Manchester UP, 2000
MacCarthy, Desmond, ed., *The Essayes of Michael Lord of Montaigne translated into English by John Florio*, I, London & Toronto, Dent, 1928
MacCulloch, Diarmaid, *Thomas Cranmer: A Life*, London & New Haven, Yale UP, 2016 edn.
Malfatti, C.V., ed., *Two Italian Accounts of Tudor England. A Journey to London in 1497*, Barcelona, C.V. Malfatti, 1953
Mancini, Dominic, *The Usurpation of Richard the Third*, ed. C.A.J. Armstrong, Gloucester, Sutton, 1989
Mead, Richard, *Short Discourse concerning Pestilential Contagion and the Methods to be used to Prevent it*, London, 1721
Mears, Natalie, and Ryrie, Alec, eds, *Worship and the Parish Church in Early Modern Britain*, London, Routledge, 2016
More, Thomas, *Utopia*, trans Paul Turner, London, Penguin, 2009
Mullett, Charles F., *The Bubonic Plague and England: An Essay in the History of Preventive Medicine*, Lexington, University of Kentucky Press, 1956
Mynors, R.A.B., Dalzell, A. and Estes, J.M., eds, *The Correspondence of Erasmus: Letters 1356 to 1534*, Toronto, University of Toronto Press, 1974 continuing
Nevinson, Charles, *Later Writings of Bishop Hooper*, Parker Soc., 1852
Nichols, J.G., ed., *Chronicle of the Grey Friars of London*, Camden Soc., 53, 1852
Nichols, J.G., ed., *The Diary of Henry Machyn Citizen and Merchant-Taylor of London (1550-1563)*, Camden Soc., 1848
Nicols, John Gough, ed., *Literary Remains of King Edward the Sixth*, I, London, Roxburghe Club, 1857
Noorthouck, John, *A New History of London Including Westminster and Southwark*, London, 1773
Norfolk: *An Essay Towards A Topographical History of the County of Norfolk: Volume 3*, London, W. Miller, 1806
Oldstone, Michael B.A., *Viruses, Plagues and History*, 2nd edn,, Oxford, OUP, 2020
Parker, Geoffrey, *Emperor: A New Life of Charles V*, London & New Haven, Yale UP, 2019
Penn, Thomas, *Winter King: The Dawn of Tudor England*, London, Penguin, 2011

Poole, H. Edmund, ed., *The Wisdom of Andrew Boorde*, Leicester, Edgar Backus, 1936

Rawcliffe, Carole, *Urban Bodies; Communal Health in Late Medieval English Towns and Cities*, Woodbridge, Boydell, 2013

Resch, Claudia, "The English Sweating Sickness' of 1529 in Augsburg: A Challenge to Body and Soul and the Printer', 2009, English abstract

Riley, H.T., *Ingulph's Chronicle of the Abbey of Croyland*, London, Henry G. Bohn, 1854

Riordan, Michael, 'Carey, William (c. 1496–1528)', *ODNB*

Robson-Scott, W.D., *German Travellers in England 1400-1800*, Oxford, Blackwell, 1953

Rodgers, Dirk W., 'À Lasco [Laski], John (1499–1560)', *ODNB*

Roger, Euan C., "To Be Shut Up': New Evidence for the Development of Quarantine Regulations in Early-Tudor England', *Social History of Medicine*, April 2019

Rogers, E.F., *St Thomas More: Selected Letters*, London & New Haven, Yale UP, 1961

Scott, Susan, and Duncan, Christopher J., *Biology of Plagues: Evidence from Historical Populations*, Cambridge, CUP, 2001

Sharpe, R.R., ed., *Calendar of Wills Proved and Enrolled in the Court of Husting, London: Part 2, 1358-1688*, London, 1890

Sharpe, Reginald R. ed., *Calendar of Letter-Books...of the City of London, L*, Corporation of London, 1912

Shrewsbury, J.F.D., *A History of Bubonic Plague in the British Isles*, Cambridge, CUP, 1970

Skeel, Caroline, *The Council in the Marches of Wales: A Study in Local Government during the Sixteenth and Seventeenth centuries*, London, H. Rees, 1904

Slack, Paul, 'The Local Incidence of Epidemic Disease: the Case of Bristol 1540-1650', *The Plague Reconsidered, Local Population Studies Supplement*, 1977

Smith, Lucy Toulmin, ed., *The Itinerary of John Leland in or about the Years 1535-1543*, London, George Bell & Son, 1907–10

Stow, John, *Annales, or a Generall Chronicle of England*, London, 1631

Stow, John, *The Survey of London*, ed. H.B. Wheatley, Dent, London, 1987

Thacker, A.T., and Lewis, C.P., eds, *A History of the County of Chester, Volume 5 Part 2, the City of Chester: Culture, Buildings, Institutions*, London, 2005

Thompson, Craig R., *Collected Works of Erasmus, Colloquies*, vol. 1, Toronto, University of Toronto Press, 1997

Thurley, Simon, *The Royal Palaces of Tudor England*, London & New Haven, Yale UP, 1993

Thurley, Simon, *Houses of Power: The Places That Shaped the Tudor World*, London, Bantam Press, 2017

Trapp, J.B., 'Ammonius, Andreas [Andrea della Rena], (bap. 1476, d. 1517)', *ODNB*

Tremlett, Chris, *Catherine of Aragon: Henry's Spanish Queen*, London, Faber & Faber, 2010

Vicary, Thomas, *The Anatomie of the Bodie of Man*, ed. Frederick J. Furnivall and Percy Furnivall, Early English Text Soc., extra series, 53, 1888

Vergil, Polydore, *The Anglica Historia 1485-1537*, in Roger Lockyer, *Henry VII*, London, Longman, 1968

Webb, Francis C., 'The Sweating Sickness in England', *The Sanitary Review and Journal of Public Health*, III, 1857

Webb, Francis C., *The Sweating Sickness in England*, London, 1857

Williams, C.H., *English Historical Documents 1485-1558*, London, Eyre & Spottiswood, 1967

Wilson, F.P., *The Plague in Shakespeare's London*, Oxford, OUP, 1927

Wrigley, E.A., and Schofield, R.S., *The Population History of England 1541-1871, A Reconstruction*, Cambridge, CUP, 1981

Wylie, J.A.H., and Collier, L.H., 'The English Sweating Sickness (sudor anglicus): a reappraisal', *Journal of the History of Medicine*, 36, 1981

Index

Act of Parliament, 33
Ammonius, Andreas, 52–4, 61
Amsterdam, 84
André, Bernard, 48
Antwerp, 80, 83–4, 112, 131
Apothecaries, 32, 34, 49
Apprentices, 56–7
D'Aragona, Luigi, 60
Arbuthnot, John, 114
Armies, 11
Arthur, Prince of Wales, 1, 43–7
Astrology, 17, 35–6
Audley, Sir Thomas, 88
Augsburg, 82

Bacon, Anthony, 104–7, 110
Bacon, Francis, 10, 110–11
Barnard's Castle, 28
Basel, 12, 36, 83–4
Bats, 121
Beaufort, Margaret, 20
Bear-baiting, 107
Becket, Thomas à, 26
Beggars, 65
Du Bellay, Jean, 7, 73–7
Bills of Mortality, 78
Black Death *see* plague
Boleyn, Anne, 70–2, 88
Boleyn, Sir Thomas, 72
Boorde, Andrew, 86–7
Bosworth, Battle of, 2, 40
Brandon, Henry and Charles, 97–9
Bremen, 81
Brewer, J. S., 117
Bridewell Palace, 28–9
Bristol, 96, 100

Broke, Richard, 74
Buckden, Huntingdonshire, 97–8
Butts, Dr William, 92

Caius, Dr John, 5–6, 34, 93–5, 110–11, 118–19
Calais, 6, 13, 52, 60, 74, 79, 120
Cambridge, 26–7, 44, 52, 54–5, 58, 96–8, 104–05, 111, 119
Campeggio, Cardinal Lorenzo, 67, 71, 77–8
Canterbury, 26–7
Carey, William, 72, 74–5
Carthusian, 24, 39, 75
Cartoons, 116
Caxton, William, 18
Cecil, William (Lord Burghley), 108
Certificates, health, 63
Chapuys, Eustace, 88
Charles I, 112–13
Charles II, 113–14
Charles V, Holy Roman Emperor, 49, 71
Charles VIII, of France, 11
Chester, 27, 43, 48, 93, 95–6
Cholmley, Sir Richard, 57
Chronicles (Raphael Holinshed), 124–31
Church's disapproval, 16–17, 83–4, 100–103
Clark, Sir George, 119
Clinton, Thomas Lord, 60
Colet, John, 53, 122
College of Physicians, Royal, 32–3
Cologne, 82, 84
Commynes, Philippe de, 2
Companies, livery, 41
Compton, Sir William, 72, 74–5

Consumption, criticism of excessive, 18–19
Copenhagen, 81
Cornwallis, Sir John, 90, 123–4
Coventry, 28, 50, 93
COVID-19, 119–22
Cranmer, Archbishop, 102
Craven, Earl of, 114
Creighton, Charles, 118
Cromwell, Thomas, 78
Croydon, 96, 102
Croyland Chronicler, 2
The Curtain playhouse, 107
Cust, Mrs Henry, 119–20

Darcy, Lord, 8
Defoe, Daniel, 36, 114
Denham, Francis, 75
Deventer, 84
DNA evidence, 16
Doctor of Physick, 32
Dogs, 16, 22, 107, 109
Dudley, Edmund, 52
Dunkirk fever, 115
Durham, 29, 96

Edmund Tudor, 43
Edward VI, 6, 89–93, 99–100, 122
Elizabeth I, 88, 104
Eltham Palace, 46, 48, 55, 69, 113
Eltham Ordinances, 74–5
Empson, Richard, 52
Enfield, 113
English Sweat *see* sweating sickness
Erasmus, Desiderius, 5–7, 12, 22–5, 33–4, 52–4
Essays (Michel de Montaigne), 106
Evil May Day riot, 56–7
Exeter, 27–8

Fairs, 65–6
Faunt, Nicholas, 104–107, 110
Ferdinand and Isabella of Spain, 44–5
Fitzroy, Henry, 29, 69, 87–8
Flanders, 6, 78
Fleas, 15–16
Florio, John, 106

Forestier, Thomas, 4–5, 23, 38–40
Foxe, John, 79–80
Foxe, Richard, 49
France, 4, 6, 11, 16–18, 53, 71–4, 77–8, 114–5
Franciscius, Andreas, 23
Frankfurt, 81, 84
Froschover, Christopher, 94, 96

Galen, 21–2
Gee, Edmund, 96
Geneva, 105
Germany, 79–83
Gigli, Giovanni and Silvetsro, 53
Giustinian, Sebastian, 56–9, 61, 67–8
Gloucester, 99
'God's punishment', 83–4
Gottfried, Robert, 119
Greenwich, 28, 48, 74, 88
Grey, Lord, of Wilton, 60–1
Greystoke, Lord John, 49
Grüner, Christianus Gottfridus, 117

Haemorrhagic fever, 82
Hall, Edward, 5, 52
Hamburg, 79–80
Hampton Court, 89–92
Hancock, Thomas, 97
Hantavirus, 1, 120–1
Hecker, J. C. D., 117
Henry VII:
  army, 2–4
  establishes Savoy hospital, 49–50
  moves away from London, 39
  pardons Forestier, 41
Henry VIII:
  birth, 50
  and chivalric pursuits, 19–20
  and music, 59
  and Katherine of Aragon, 44–7, 70–1, 77–8, 87
  and Anne Boleyn, 70–1, 87
  breaks with Rome, 78
  and Jane Seymour, 88–9
  J. S. Brewer's *Letters and Papers*, 117
Herd, John, 102
Hereford, Herefordshire, 16

Hever Castle, 72
Hill, Mayor Sir Thomas, 3, 38, 41–2
The History of England (David Hume), 116
Holinshed, Raphael, 100, 103, 111–12, 128–31
Hooper, Bishop John, 99, 102
Hospitals, 27, 42, 50
Household Orders of 1539, 123–7
Houses, infected, markings, 63–6
Hubertus, Thomas, 6, 81, 119
Hull, 97
Hustings, Court of, 41

In Praise of Folly (Erasmus), 33–4
Influenza, 102–3, 119–20
Inner Temple, The, 55, 60
Insects, 121
Italian plague regulations, 62–3
Italy, 4, 11, 16, 32, 54, 62, 108

James I, 112
Jones, John, 103
A Journal of the Plague Year (Defoe), 36
Jousts and tournaments, 19, 129

Katherine of Aragon, 44–7, 70–1, 77–8

Laski, Jan, 102
Leland, John, 27
Leprosy, 12
Linacre, Thomas, 32
Lincoln, Bishop of, 72, 98
Lisle, Lord and Lady, 87–8
London, 25–6
    Lord Mayor, 106, 108
    social conditions in, 23–4
    see also under individual districts
Loughborough, 95, 97, 119
Ludlow, 44–7, 93
Luther, Martin, 82
Lyly, John, 7

Machyn, Henry, 93
Malaria, 92
Maler, Josua, 99
Mancini, Dominic, 27

Marburg Articles, 82
Markets, 21, 24, 26, 44, 58, 66
Mary Tudor, Princess, 69
Mayerne, Theodore de, 114
Mead, Richard, 114–15
Memo, Dionysius, 59–60, 73
Merchants, 25–6, 53–62, 79, 93
Milan, 108
Montaigne, Michel de, 106
The More Palace, 31
More, Thomas, 5, 18–19, 21, 65
Mountjoy, Lord, 52

Neapolitan sickness, 11
The Netherlands, 84
Nonsuch Palace, 31, 113
Noorthouck, John, 4
Norfolk, Countess of, 76
Norfolk, Elizabeth Duchess of, 5–8
Norwich, 27, 43, 47, 96

Orders, enforcement, 108–109, 123–7
Oxford, 3, 26–7, 58, 65, 99, 113

Palaces, royal, 28
    see also under individual palaces
Pamphlets, 82–3
Paris, 66, 70, 105
Pesthouses, 107
Physicians, 32–3, 49, 109, 111
Picardy Sweat, 4, 114
Pilgrimages, 86
Plague, 13–14, 54–68, 92–3, 113–14
Plays, 107–9
Poor Clares at the Minories, 55–6
Portugal, 85
Pox, French, 11, 17
Poyntz, Sir Francis, 72
Proclamation, Royal (1518), 64–6
Procopius, 14
Prostitutes, 112
Prussia, 81

Quarantine, 62–4, 107–109

Richard III, 2
Richmond, Duke of, 75

Richmond Palace, 28, 39, 48, 69, 99
Rodents, 121
Rods, white, 63–5
Royal court, size of, 30–1
Russell, Sir John, 87
Russia, 14, 81
Rutland, Lady, 89
Ryff, Fridolin, 84

St Anthony's crosses, 92, 107
St Paul's, 3, 40, 48, 53, 55–6
St Roch, 117
St Sebastian, 17
Salisbury, 31, 113
Savorgnano, Mario, 27
Savoy hospital, 50
Scandinavia, 14, 81
Seymour, Jane, 88–90
Shakespeare, William, 4
Sheen Palace *see* Richmond Palace
Sheriff Hutton, 75, 87
Shoreditch, 3, 107
Shrewsbury (plane name), 93-4, 130
Shrewsbury, Earl of, 56, 117
Shrewsbury, J. F. D., 119
Sidney, Sir William, 90
Simeon, Geoffrey, 49
Sloane, Sir Hans, 114
Soranzo, Giacomo, 5, 27, 102–103
Spain, 25-6, 45, 49, 72-3, 85, 130
Stanley, Lord, 2–3
Stokker, Mayor Sir William, 3
Stopgallant sweat *see* sweating sickness
Stow, John, 47, 93–4
Strasburg, 82
Sudor Anglicus see sweating sickness
Summers, Henry, 75
Sumptuary legislation, 19
Surgeons, 12, 33
Sweating sickness:
  start of outbreak, 38
  name, 1, 6
  identification, failure of, 1–2
  origins, 2–4
  symptoms, 4–6
  death rates, 6, 38–40, 77–8, 93–6, 100

nursing care, 7–9
medicines, 8–9
spreads into Europe, 79–85
on the continent, 6, 114–16
and younger men, 97–8, 112
and church's disapproval, 100–104
modern studies, 119–22
Syon House, 99, 113

The Theatre playhouse, 107
Travellers, movement of, 24–7
Tudor, Henry *see* Henry VII
Tuke, Sir Brian, 6, 10, 35, 76, 78–9
Tyndale, William, 79–80
Typhus, 120
Tyttenhanger, 31, 73–4

Universities, 3, 17, 26, 54, 75
Urban infilling, 27–8

Venice, 25, 35, 59-61, 67, 71, 77
Ventilation in houses, 24–5
Vergil, Polydore, 4, 7, 53
Vienna, 83

Waldstein, Baron, 30
Walshingham Priory, 86
Warbeck, Perkin, 44
Webb, Francis, 116
Westminster, 29, 87, 110
Whitehall Palace, 29–30
Wills, 41–3, 75, 80
Winchester, 27, 31, 70
Winchester, Bishop of, 29, 49, 58, 88
Windsor, 59–60, 64, 74, 87–8
Wingfield, Sir Richard, 60
Wolsey, Cardinal Thomas, 22, 29, 77–8
Worcester, 28, 43
Wych, Dame Alice, 12

Yersinia pestis, 15–16
York, 27–9, 43, 50, 97
York Place, 29–31

Zwingli, Ulrich, 82